AF333630

deadly medicine

deadly medicine

DOCTORS AND TRUE CRIME

Arthur Kent

Taplinger Publishing Company | New York

First published in the United States in 1975 by
TAPLINGER PULISHING CO., INC.
New York, New York

Published in the United Kingdom in 1974 as *The Death Doctors*.

Library of Congress Catalog Card Number: 74-20210

ISBN 0-8008-2129-7

AUTHOR'S NOTE

In my researches for the material in THE DEATH DOCTORS, I was forced to rely, in the main, on newspaper accounts of trials, because many of the American and French cases have not yet been given a more permanent, and easily accessible, treatment in book form.

The toxicological history, which is a sub-theme in the book, has been covered in a more general and technical sense in PROOF OF POISON by Jürgen Thorwald, which also deals with the fight to establish a good name for toxicology over the last hundred and fifty years. Also of assistance to me were BERNARD SPILSBURY (HIS LIFE AND CASES) by Douglas G. Browne and E. V. Tullett, (George G. Harrap, 1952), and ENCYCLO-PAEDIA OF MURDER by Colin Wilson and Pat Pitman, (Arthur Barker, 1961).

The careers of doctors such as Smethurst, Pritchard and Crippen have been well documented in NOTABLE BRITISH TRIALS, the series published in Scotland by William Hodge & Company, to which readers can turn for full accounts of their careers. Unhappily, there are no such comparable works in the United States or France for further studies into the lives of such mass murderers as Dr. Holmes or Dr. Petiot.

A.K.

CONTENTS

INTRODUCTION

Nobody could have realized at the time, but 1823 was a watershed year for the medical profession, for it was then that the first doctor was caught out in murder through poison being detected inside his victim's body. At last, after centuries, post mortems had begun to tell the lurid truth.

With the arrest of Dr. Edme Castaing in 1823, poisoners must have realized that the golden years of poisoning without any legal comeback, had gone forever. If the authorities could catch out a doctor, an expert on medicines, what chance did they have as laymen?

Before the first tentative steps into toxicology and medical jurisprudence made by doctors in Sweden, Germany, England and France, poisoners had had a clear run. The Cesare Borgias and the Marie Brinvilliers had blithely and confidentally peddled Spouse-remover and Inheritance-powder by the wholesale ton. Just occasionally, a poisoner came a cropper; but this had invariably been brought about by carelessness in the purchase of the powder or because bribery, torture, or conscience had made an accomplice talk.

Arsenic had been the customary powder. It had many advantages. It was tasteless and colourless and odourless. It blended nicely with delicate broths and heavy stews, and the symptoms of illness didn't arouse suspicion because they were similar to cholera which was rampant across Europe. But with the advent of toxicology and the ability to find cause of death by making tests *within* the body, poisoners had to think again. Arsenic, an irritant metallic poison, became easy to spot.

Poisoners were forced to turn to poisons which were hard to detect, and leading them, as experts, were the doctors. They turned to vegetable drugs and chemicals, and there were hundreds to choose from – morphine had been isolated from opium, strychnine from nux vomica, caffeine from coffee, and so on.

Three doctors, of which Dr. Castaing was the first, tried unsuccessfully in the nineteenth century to out-fox the medical inquiry that might follow the death of their victims by a cunning blending of drugs or by going outside the known ranges. I mention them in the introduction because I have not included their stories in the book, giving the space instead to the activities of more fascinating murdering practitioners.

Dr. Castaing murdered with panache and a conviction that his method would never be discovered. He used morphine on two friends. They were the brothers Ballet. Hippolyte Ballet, who was wealthy, was slow in dying from consumption and his brother, Auguste, asked Castaing to give him a lethal kick on his way so that he could inherit his money. Dr. Castaing agreed, providing Auguste would write a will favouring him. Trustingly, Auguste did, and six months after Hippolyte died, Auguste followed him.

As Auguste was dying, he asked Castaing to call in another doctor and, without a qualm, Castaing did. The doctor who arrived called in yet another expert – and both noticed a narrowing of the pupils of Auguste's eyes, which is now recognized as a symptom of morphine poisoning. (Later in the book, you will read how the American doctor, Robert Buchanan, successfully got round this betraying factor).

When Castaing informed his colleagues that he would inherit Auguste's fortune, they immediately suggested that he should avoid scandal and gossip by calling for a post mortem. As a result, morphine was found in the body, but medical experts couldn't agree at Castaing's trial whether it was in sufficient amounts to kill. However, the jury, much to Castaing's surprise, accepted secondary circumstantial evidence which indicated that Auguste had died as a result of morphine poisoning. Their verdict was based on evidence of the narrowing of the pupils, vomiting, fatigue, and paralysis of the central nervous system. Castaing went to the guillotine.

In Paris, also, Dr. Couty de la Pommerais committed two murders during the 1860's. For the first he used digitalis, which gave the same symptoms as cholera, which, until then, could not be detected in the body. With this drug, Dr. de la Pommerais murdered his wife, who left him a fortune, and this not being enough, he then murdered his mistress, after persuading her to take out insurance in his favour. Suspicion against him, however, was so strong that the authorities told their doctors to try every method possible to find poison in the bodies of the wife and mistress. They persevered and experimented – and they detected, so another doctor went to the guillotine.

Despite the many casualties to the public executioner, there were other challengers, including Dr. George Lampson, of England, who poisoned his brother-in-law for the few hundred pounds of a possible inheritance. He came back from the United

States with some empty capsules, which had been invented to make the absorption of medicine more palatable, and filled one of them with aconitine and sugar, which he administered to his brother-in-law. Lampson stood trial at the Old Bailey in 1882. Medical evidence didn't wholly prove, however, that his victim had died of aconitine, but the other evidence, such as the purchase of the drug by him, satisfied the jury of his guilt and he was hanged.

It is not the intention in this work to go too deeply into the complex and technical history of toxicology, but for readers who would like to know more about this aspect of it, I would strongly recommend PROOF OF POISON by Jürgen Thorwald, which was published by Thames and Hudson in 1966.

What the Castaing affair in Paris proved was not only that medical jurisprudence was able to detect poison in a victim, but could do so in the victim of a medically-qualified doctor who was using his skill cunningly. But, as some of the stories in this work will indicate, there were medical setbacks in court, conflict and controversy with medical testimony of an unhappy kind, and of a kind which still exists today.

Medicine isn't an exact science. For every medical expert who would say in court that the deceased had been scuppered by poison, another would call it death by natural wastage. Even so, the Castaing trial was a triumph for toxicology.

But, ironically, what the medical profession was doing in exposing their murdering colleagues, was getting the entire profession a bad name. In the nineteenth century, the man in the street was alarmed by the seemingly large numbers of doctors who were standing trial as killers. Worse, it seemed that they were trying by every cunning means to out-fox the toxicologists by using drugs which couldn't be detected at post mortems. Can we blame the Victorian if he pondered the question of how many doctors there were around who might be getting away with murder? It looked as if only the cocksure and the clumsy were being apprehended. As some of these cases show, the entire affair seemed to have taken on the proportions of a macabre parlour game in which the murdering English, American and French doctor called on his lethal resources to outwit the doctors fielded against him by the authorities.

Doctors, with murder in their minds, weren't slow in learning from the mistakes of their brethren who had already been exposed and executed. Dr. Pritchard realized that Dr. Palmer had been caught out because his victim died too quickly after being known to be in good health. So he used small doses on his wife so that she lingered in illness over several months before he gave her the final killing dose. In New York, Dr. Buchanan saw the medical student, Carlyle Harris, go to the electric chair because he hadn't attempted to disguise his use of morphine, and so he found a way to murder by the same method so – he hoped – the drug wouldn't show. All murder is, of course, evil but murder by poison is more reprehensible than any other method. It has been described as the weapon of women. It is certainly the weapon of the weak and little man – and, strangely, so many of the doctors named in this work were little men, physically, as well as in character. But even so, poison does have an overwhelming advantage over the blunt instrument. It leaves no signs of violence. If the poisoner has done his homework well and has not been clumsy, he stands a good chance of having the death labelled as due to natural causes. Especially, as so often happened, he signed the death certificate himself.

Perhaps, theoretically, these doctors could be excused for using drugs where other poisoners could not, for, as most killers will, they were only turning to the weapon they knew best.

What most surprised me in my researches, was the large number of doctors who turned to murder. It seemed as if murder was an affliction of the profession in much the way silicosis was a hazard in the mining industry. I would be hard put to it, I am sure, to find a comparable number of lawyers, soldiers, clergymen, butchers, bakers and candlestick makers who had killed wives, relatives and neighbours. It is also true to say that in several instances Victorian rectitude was the spur for murder. If divorce had been cheap and easy, and had carried with it no social disgrace, some of the doctors mentioned here, wouldn't be here. The need for a facade of respectability had equal strength with their sexual appetites, and their wives just had to go. But yet other doctors here just murdered for the fun of it, and some on a massive scale.

Because of their activities, the medical profession carried a bad name in Victorian times, and this was sad since it was the period when the birth of modern medicine began. While the DEATH DOCTORS were carrying out their mass slaughters, Joseph Lister, unnoticed, was discovering antiseptics; Smith and Simon were evolving sanitation and a scheme for public health which would eradicate diseases such as cholera; and Wright and Addison were identifying diseases.

If, statistically, doctors appear to have murdered by poison more than any other group, it is perhaps because they have been tempted by the poison cupboard being only a few yards away. After all, there are a large number of people killed and injured in the United States each year by firearms, but then every neighbourhood has its friendly gunsmith at the corner. Perhaps because doctors have a God-like power to save life, and do so in great numbers, some of them are tempted at times to take the same God-like right and take a few lives. Jungle habits do die hard.

The Victorian legal expert, Sir James Stephen, was sardonically amused by the shock occasioned when a doctor of poise and polish faced trial for murder by poison. Stephen said, "The case supplies proof – which kind-hearted people seem to doubt – that wickedness is inconsistent with good education, perfect sanity and everything which deprives men of an excuse to commit murder." True then, probably more true now. No century has had more knowledge and more education and more comfort than the twentieth century, yet no century has seen as much violence. No nation produces, on average, more charming and eloquent people than Ireland, but very few modern countries could have known such civic strife. Still, for some of the educated, the sword still speaks more sharply than the written and spoken word.

With the exception of the American, Dr. Hermann Sander, who was found not guilty of killing a patient, all the doctors in this work were criminals. Dr. Sander is the odd man out, the hero, and by his suffering has shown the despair a doctor often feels in his fight to save life and suffering. But both Dr. Smethurst and Dr. Knox deserve a modicum of compassion. Their guilt wasn't proven beyond all doubt.

Arthur Kent

DR. ROBERT KNOX

Up the close and down the stair
Around the house with Burke and Hare
Burke's the butcher, Hare's the thief,
Knox the boy who buys the beef.

This jingle which went the rounds in Scotland in 1829 and was
to horrify generations of Scots as yet unborn, concerned the
gruesome activities of William Burke and William Hare who
murdered some sixteen friends and acquaintances in order to
keep Dr. Robert Knox supplied with bodies for dissection in his
anatomy classes. Burke was to hang, Hare to escape (after turning witness for the state), and Dr. Knox, a brilliant surgeon,
rightly or wrongly, to be hounded all his life for his part in the
ghastly affair.

A teacher, no matter how brilliant, is only as good as his tools
and equipment would allow him to be and Dr. Knox, probably
the best anatomist among the half a dozen or so surgeons teaching anatomy in Edinburgh in the 1820s, needed a never-ending
supply of cadavers for his classes – classes which held more pupils
than his rivals and convened more often, because his fame had
gone before him. Dr. Knox consequently, on occasions, found
himself with a packed class of eager students but no body on the
slab for dissection.

Anatomists hadn't always been so badly treated. The rule had
been that the bodies of executed criminals should be sent to the
anatomists. This had worked well enough in the centuries which
had gone before, when executions were common and anatomists
few; but when Dr. Knox began his teaching, executions had
become rarer and there were more anatomists demanding bodies.
Whenever there is a demand for something there is always a
few adventurous spirits on hand to step forward and create a
business. Thus people soon heard whispers of a new, secret
professional body of men – the ressurectionists. In Edinburgh
and London body-snatching from cemeteries became a nightly
happening and a decried scandal. Dr. Knox alone needed seventy

fresh bodies a year, each of which was only sufficient for several lessons, and he was only one recipient of the regular suppliers.

With Edinburgh University high on surgery and low on ethics, it is easy to imagine, human nature being what it was, what must eventually happen. Somebody with a little more neck than his neighbour would soon be poaching bodies on the streets, after delivering a more than playful tap on the cranium.

Along with the professional resurrectionists, were bodies of students who raided churchyards as a prank – a prank which also brought profit. The winter rate for a body in prime condition was £10, the summer rate £8, as much money as a labourer would earn in hard toil in as many weeks. The church authorities and families took what precautions they could. Guards were placed at cemeteries during the night, and in larger establishments watch towers and patrols were used. But resurrectionists, proud of their trade, boasted of their successes. It was said they could sneak into a cemetery, remove the fresh dirt from a new grave, prise off the coffin lid, drag the corpse out by its neck, and have everything back in its place in minutes. Because it was a criminal offence to steal a shroud, but not a body, the shroud would be left behind, and the naked body carried off in a sack. Consequently another name for the resurrectionists became "the sack-'em-up-men". Some resurrectionists used a heavy grapple which ripped the lid off the coffin. No matter what precautions were taken, the resurrectionists claimed they could circumnavigate them.

Dr. Knox began teaching in Edinburgh in 1822. Although considered a brilliant teacher, he had a forbidding manner and unattractive appearance and made enemies easily. He had a gaunt, cadverous-like presence. An attack of smallpox had cost him the sight of one eye and earned him the nickname of Doctor Cyclops. Caustic of tongue, a dandy in his dress, he nevertheless soon became a hero with his pupils. An eye-witness left the following word-picture of Dr. Knox conducting a class:

> "When Knox sat down to instruct a pupil it was in a masterly fashion; the fine sweep of the scalpel, the line of precision, the unfolding of tissues, and finally a clear demonstration with a fund of information, physiological, surgical and pathological. When he saw a pupil slashing away at the muscles of a part, he touched the young man's shoulder and said, 'Ah, sir! I see you are dissecting for the sake of the bones. Wouldn't it be as well to pick up a few facts as to the attachments and uses of these muscles before you reach the skeleton'?"

But if a hero to his pupils, Knox was disliked outside Surgeons Square. He had married secretly, "a person of inferior rank", it was said, and for this he was criticized first by one section (for being a snob), and then by another for not showing his wife openly. Moreover his politics, said to be radical, were out of tune with the times. Knox was both malicious and callous. He began a lecture one day by smirkingly telling his pupils: "I hear that Doctor Robert Liston has mistaken an aneurism for an abcess and lanced it. I take it none of you are too dumb to know what that means. It means the patient's dead."

When the scandal of the Burke and Hare murders broke, therefore, and it was discovered that sixteen freshly-dead victims had been hurried from the place of violence to Dr. Knox's rooms, his colleagues were among the first to ask awkward questions.

What gave Burke and Hare an advantage over the conventional grave-robbers (and would have told in their favour if it had suddenly become a buyer's market), was the fact that their corpses were always fresh. You could rightly say *picked this morning*. They certainly didn't suggest in any way that they had been purloined from graves, which would mean they were several days old. The corpses that the Burke & Hare firm were delivering to Knox in an efficient and steady stream had obviously died, and mysteriously so, some few hours before. And yet Dr. Knox, excited by their sweetness, never questioned the pair. In most cases the bodies would have shown, in a post mortem, some indication that they had died by violence. Yet Dr. Knox, who was dissecting these victims with the aid of his students, never seems to have discovered what had killed them. And the appearance of Burke & Hare, arriving in the anonymity of night with their sacked up wares, was enough to create suspicions in a saint. But all the pair got from Knox and his assistants was approval, delight at the corpses freshness, and encouragement to keep the supplies coming.

The two murderers, a couple of not-too-bright nineteenth century spivs, came on the business by accident. William Hare (with a widow named Maggie Laird) was running a cheap doss-house in Tanners Close. It was so cheap that you slept under sacking on a straw-covered floor. William Burke, who had been born in County Tyrone, Ireland, came and lodged there with his common law wife, a prostitute named Helen McDougal. Burke described himself as a dancing master but, in fact, made a precarious living repairing shoes. His laziness heightened this precariousness, although Edinburgh had been going through a gradually worsening slump since the end of the Napoleonic wars.

When Hare and his lodger were in funds they were invariably drunk with their women. When without, they were invariably dreaming and scheming on how they might get a dram. On a dry day a Highlander known as Old Donald keeled over and died and Maggie, with no spirit to keep her warm, bemoaned (loudly) that the old soldier had gone before he could pick up his quarterly army pension and still owed her £4. The four reflected dumbly on the tragedy of it all when one of them piped up and suggested they "flog" him to Dr. Knox in order to get Maggie recompensed. A neighbour, David Paterson, worked as porter for Dr. Knox and probably had dropped the hint from time to time to the penniless pair that they should find a corpse or two and peddle it to his master.

A coffin had already been ordered for Old Donald. But thirst makes minds work faster. This problem was overcome by the box being filled with bark, and the bark went one way for burial and Old Donald went the other way for dissection in a sack. The shifty-eyed pair, perspiring some, dealt with three of Dr. Knox's assistants at his rooms in Surgeon's Square. They were William Fergusson, Thomas Jones and Alexander Miller – all to be famous surgeons eventually. The students minutely inspected the corpse and were delighted by its freshness, a point mentally recorded by the pair. Because they were ill at ease however, it seemed they were robbed, and only received £7 10s, instead of the usual rate.

But they were delighted. Usually they had to slog hard for an entire week to earn £1 at labouring, and during the celebration which followed, their tongues loosened, thoughts and ambitions flying high, they must surely have speculated about the future with their womenfolk. Perhaps it was suggested that they become resurrectionists, sack-'em-up-men, but neither Burke nor Hare were of the stuff of which ressurectionists are made. It was a dangerous profession. Cemeteries were now guarded at night by armed men who didn't hesitate to shoot. Much better to poach the corpses before they got to their last resting place. And by now there were already too many sack-'em-up-men chasing too few bodies around the Edinburgh cemeteries. There was such a shortage of bodies, in fact, that a thriving import industry was underway, and Irish bodies were being shipped from Dublin in crates labelled *piano*, *books* and *animals for museums*.

Murder wasn't yet in the Burke and Hare curriculum. Like most business's theirs developed by slow step following slow step and by improvization. They speculated on the prospects that more of their lodgers might die, and on this first occasion, probably went no further than deciding that they might only take in lodgers who looked, so to speak, as if they were on their last legs. And so it came about that the second cadaver presented itself. It was a sort of half-murder because the second prospect, unlike the first, needed a little nudge to help him on his way.

They had liked the nice look of the lodger, named Joseph, when they first saw him. Hare suspected cholera, and thought if word got out that a man was down with fever, it would be bad for dosshouse business. Burke thought poor old Joe looked bad and something should be done to ease his suffering. When he came out of a coma, they poured whisky down his gullet. When the shock didn't kill him, Hare held him down while Burke helped him to stop breathing by pressing a pillow over his face. Either Joe was more delectable or the pair were more confident and businesslike, or Knox, delighted with the freshness of their wares, had told his assistants to give them prime prices, for this time they picked up £10. But it was Christmas, an expensive time, and with Hogmanay close behind, they were soon broke. And now they took to the streets. It must have been a frustrating month for them, with many comic touches, as they searched the mean streets of West Port looking for prospects. Following an old drab here and a drunk there, hoping the prospect might drop dead, but both drawing back at the last moment, too frightened to give a knockout punch when he didn't collapse like they hoped he would.

But a shortage in the purse gave a fillip to their courage. On February 11, they picked up an ancient crone named Abigail Simpson, who lived on a small pension and who peddled salt. She had just collected her 18 pence dole and was drinking it in a tavern, when smiling Burke and cheerful Hare, touring the taverns for prospects, joined her in the bar. She was drunk – and she had no friends or relatives. They insisted she return to the dosshouse with them for a wee dram.

Abigail was plied with more drink until she was senseless. Her flimsy hands and legs were firmly held by Burke while Hare covered her nose and mouth and smothered her. The pair sent word to Surgeon's Square that *John* and *William* would be round that night with another fresh subject. Abigail was taken on her last journey folded into a tea chest. It was to be a special occasion. Dr. Knox was there to meet them. The fact that he himself was on hand at such a late hour, and after he must have heard that the pair were arriving with a body, is worth considering. It might of course have been pure chance, as no doubt his defenders would say it was. But it could equally have been the wish to see *John* and *William* who were something different in the sack-'em-up business in that they produced fresh-this-morning corpses, and not the partially decayed, stiffening, grave-soiled goods of other resurrectionists.

Dr. Knox inspected Abigail himself. He commented on how fresh she was and was obviously pleased by this fact. He didn't ask any awkward questions but promptly paid over £10, and showed the men the door. It is said in Dr. Knox's defence, and with some justification, that anatomists had adopted the practice of never asking questions of resurrectionists lest they frighten them away, which would mean that rival anatomists would get the business. Be that as it may, the fact is that Burke and Hare, neither of whom were morally courageous, certainly received encouragement from Dr. Knox on this evening, and it seems to have been more than a financial reward. Dr. Knox must have suspected something to be wrong yet he gave the illiterate scoundrels a moral endorsement, one which they would have prized as much as the money, because it came from somebody who was eminent and far above them socially, financially and educationally. Might they not even have assumed, for they were grossly stupid, that Knox was giving them the go-ahead, and that if the truth came out he would come forward and make it right? It could well have been. The pair certainly showed a heightened confidence after their meeting with the doctor. The whisky was flowing now at the dosshouse and the couples brought flamboyant gewgaws and became the envy of the mean streets.

They explained their wealth by hinting at an inheritance which was coming by instalments from the country, and when they were running short and others were present, they would remind each other with a nod and a wink that they must write off to the country for more funds. This was the code for them that Dr. Knox was waiting for a side of *beef*. Burke let it be known that he was a resurrectionist. This made him a hero in the taverns, especially as he was buying the drinks, and with great expectations arriving, Helen was above common whoring.

An English match-peddler was the next victim. He went down with jaundice at the dosshouse and again the excuse was that they were preserving the house's trade and good name. Hare held his kicking legs while Burke suffocated him, his own improvisation this, by gripping his nose and mouth. He was followed by an old woman enticed into the house by free drinks. The killers weren't sufficiently interested to discover the names of these victims. The next victim was important in several respects. She was an attractive and popular young prostitute named Mary Paterson, who would certainly be missed. Burke met Mary and another whore in a tavern after a night of drinking and invited them home for breakfast. His interest, at first, seemed to have been amatory and not anatomical, for he took them to the house of his brother, Constantine, who had no idea where the money was coming from. Burke got his brother's family up and making breakfast, while he gave liberally of the whisky bottle. Mary went into a tipsy sleep and Burke took the other girl, Janet Brown, to a nearby tavern for beer and pies. He returned to the house and was having his will with one or both of the girls, when Helen McDougal crashed into the house and started a scene. Janet, fortunately for her, left; Mary slept on. One thing led to another for Burke. In order to excuse himself he told Helen that his only interest in the whore was business. A wink and a nudge and Helen understood. Hare arrived, Mary was suffocated, and Helen was pacified. Fornication, not murder, was the cardinal sin.

But Mary Paterson was to give them a few headaches at the time and would help, eventually, to add to the damage done to Dr. Knox's name. It began for the killers when they carried Mary, in a sack, through the streets to Surgeon's Square. Some boys, recognizing a body by the shape of the sack, ran after them screaming.

"Hey," they yelled to a passerby, "they've got a body in the sack."

Sweating and cursing, the frightened killers had to put down the corpse to cuff and drive away the urchins. Another shock waited for them at the doctor's room, where his assistants, forewarned, waited. Two students, William Fergusson and Alexander Miller, recognized the corpse. It transpired that one of them had used her services only a night or two before. Then she had been full of the joys of life and now, suddenly, she was dead. They plied the killers with questions. They answered that they had brought the body from an old lady behind the Canongate. Both students noticed that the body was still warm. David Paterson, the porter, would write later, (aided by a ghost writer). "The beautiful symmetry and freshness of the body attracted my attention immediately." He added pompously, and in order to show that he was public spirited, that his curiosity and suspicions were aroused so much, that he was determined to question the pair when they next arrived with a body. It seems he never did, and that if he did, his intentions were to get a share of the money.

Dr. Knox was delighted with Mary Paterson. The beauty of the young body impressed him as much as the freshness. The students expressed their concern, told the doctor who the girl was, and that she had been seen a day or so before in the streets, alive and well. It seems that Dr. Knox brushed all these issues aside. He was so delighted by Mary's beautiful form, it appears, that he decided not to dissect her. After all, she would bring the young male students flocking. It wasn't expressed as indecorously as that of course. But Dr. Knox decided that she would be pickled in whisky and brought out at sessions (on muscular-control and development) so that her body could be studied. Even after death Mary's body had to work, and she wasn't dissected for three months.

A student named Henry Lonsdale, who attended the school at the time, later recorded:

> "The body of the girl couldn't fail to attract attention by its volumptous form and beauty. Students crowded around the table and artists came to study a model of Philias. Here was publicity (for the doctor and the school) beyond the professional walk. A pupil who had been in her company only a few nights before, stood aghast on observing the beautiful Lias stretched in death and ready for the scalpel."

Unknowingly, Burke and Hare had introduced something new – a freshness – into the resurrection business. Dr. Knox hadn't received such a flow of new corpses since the occasional fruits of the gallows had come to his dissecting table. *He* wasn't asking questions but the student who had been with Mary Paterson, spurred no doubt by a youthful romanticism, had demanded to know how they had got the body. Glibly the pair had offered to take him to the house where they had purchased her. They implied that drink and a lack of food had killed the girl. Since there was a tendency for prostitutes to die in this manner, and the body smelt of liquor, the student had accepted the fact. Dr. Knox certainly didn't lose a moment's sleep.

But like with most fledging businesses, there were problems at the dosshouse. Disputes and clashes of personality developed between the directors, pertaining to future policy and direction. Burke went off to the country for a few days, either for a holiday or to see about opening a district office. In his absence, Hare despatched a victim and collected on him by himself, which caused some jealousy and, (no doubt), a feeling of vulnerability on Burke's part. The women argued. Maggie didn't like Helen and dropped helpful hints that she should be taken in a sack to Knox. But in the main, Burke and Hare got on well together. They were closer than brothers. Eventually, when they tried to go their separate ways, they discovered they couldn't function efficiently. They could only do well together.

Next the pair brought off a double murder, a mother and her son. The mother was a beggar, the boy a dumb mute. The pair offered them food and rest in the dosshouse. Burke first strangled the mother and then broke the back of the boy. They were then delivered in a herring box to Dr. Knox for £16. There was a grim moment of comedy in this journey, for they hired an ancient horse to drag the box to Surgeon's Square. The horse became neurotic in the busy Grassmarket and refused under threats, kicks and the whip to move. A porter had to be hired to help with the box and, to get revenge, the pair slit the horse's throat.

Burke's holiday produced a cousin of Helen's named Anne, who was invited to the city for a visit. But Burke showed sensitivity here by asking Hare to smother her, because she was almost family. So Hare carried out the execution.

After Mary Paterson, the most famous of their victims, and again a victim who damaged Knox, was a celebrated character around Edinburgh named Daft Jamie. Everybody liked the half-witted boy who would be given lodgings and food in any part of the city where he had finished up in his wanderings by nightfall. If anybody should have made Dr. Knox pause, hesitate, wonder and investigate, it was the fresh corpse of Daft Jamie arriving at his door.

Daft Jamie was immediately recognized by the students when he was dumped on the table from the Burke and Hare sack. Not only was he recognized but some manner of his dying was indicated by blood and bruising. The crippled boy had unexpected strength and had put up a fierce fight for his life; kicking, punching, scratching. Violence certainly showed on his face, chest and legs, but Dr. Knox apparently ignored these signs and also the doubts raised by his assistants. But he must have realized the seriousness of his position for he dissected the body at his first session the next morning. A student said with horror, "Why, sir, that's Daft Jamie!" Denying it was so, Dr. Knox went briskly on with his lecture, and the dissection.

Burke and Hare were arrested after the murder of a crone on Hallowe'en. She was named Dochetty, and the gruesome-twosome had to first hide her body from two of the dosshouse's lodgers, a couple named Grey. But the Greys returned prematurely, were suspicious, and they soon found Dochetty buried in the straw with her face bloody. There came several macabrely comic scenes as Helen and Maggie unsuccessfully tried to quieten and bribe the Greys, while the men hustled the corpse, by a tortuous route, to Surgeon's Square before the police arrived. It was as if the men assumed they would be in the clear once Knox had taken delivery of the *beef*. When the police called at Knox's for the body, the doctor threatened them from the upstairs room with a pistol. He refused to let them in, and they were forced to break down the front door.

The doctors who carried out the post mortem on Dochetty found bruising, but couldn't decide whether this was criminal or had accidentally been caused when the woman might have fallen about while drunk. While the evidence was indicative of violence and even murder, it could be explained away as accidental. But things looked black for Knox, who had taken delivery of at least sixteen bodies killed in a like manner. If violence showed on this corpse, it was argued, then it would have shown on all the others. How could Knox receive so many bruised bodies from one source without asking questions or taking his suspicions to the authorities? These were the questions people were soon asking.

At least two victims, Mary Paterson and Daft Jamie, were young. They were well-known and when seen in the streets just prior to their arrival as fresh corpses at the surgery, were healthy. Yet both had brought no questions from Knox when they arrived on his dissecting table. Rather, the doctor had parried questions. Both had died in the same mysterious manner and yet Knox, seemingly, hadn't been professionally or humanly curious enough to want to discover how they had died. Dr. Knox wasn't questioned. Nor was he called to give evidence at the trial of Burke. Hare saved his own life and won his freedom by informing against Burke, who was the only one of the four dosshouse inhabitants to die on the gallows.

Dr. Knox was soon left alone in Edinburgh to face the abuse and the threats from the angry public. He defended himself by largely ignoring public opinion with his usual arrogance, but also with a display of courage. His surgery was stoned, he was lampooned in print, he was ignored in polite society and ostracized at his clubs. There was a cry for a public investigation into his activities, but none came. Leading the attack against him was the press, and the *Caledonian Mercury* reported:

> "With regard to Dr. Knox, too much delicacy and reserve have been maintained by a part of the press. It is stated that Knox conducted himself with the utmost civility to the police who went to the house in search of Dochetty's body. But the fact is he swore at them from his window and threatened to blow their brains out. It was only on their forcing the door that it was opened by one of the keepers.
> "Great pains, too, have been taken to persuade the public that the doctor was imposed upon by Burke and Hare with regard to the mode in which they acquired their subjects. But mark how a few queries will put down that supposition. Were not the bodies – one of them a girl with her hair *en papillote* – both warm and supple, repeatedly received into

his lecture room? Didn't Burke and Hare exclusively deal with Dr. Knox, and must not all their subjects have exhibited nearly the same symptoms as in the case of Dochetty, which satisfied other medical men that she had been violently bereaved of life? And why didn't the constant recurrence of these symptoms, as well as the symptoms themselves, rouse Dr. Knox's suspicion?"

Knox's porter, David Paterson, who later left the doctor's employment, said he was under instructions from Knox not to press resurrectionists too closely on where they had obtained bodies, lest they take fright and take future *beef* elsewhere. Paterson also said that it was the doctor's custom to dissect the oldest bodies first but he had made an exception with Daft Jamie, both because the boy had been recognized by a student and because, a popular figure, the boy would soon be missed in the streets.

Throughout the uproar, trial and execution of Burke, Knox continued to live and lecture as much as he had before. His students were solidly behind him and it was because of their unswerving loyalty, then and later, that little is known about what happened when Burke and Hare arrived with so many fresh bodies. Dr. Knox declined to sue his many detractors for libel or slander. He said, in one of his rare utterances on the matter:

> "The public will never understand for the most innocent proceedings even in the best conducted dissecting room must always shock. A shocked public would be hurtful of science."

An unofficial committee looked into Knox's activities. Sir Walter Scott refused to serve on it and the public were violently against it, claiming, wrongly, that it was packed with Knox's friends. The committee cleared the doctor of any criminality because, they said, his open manner and the fact that he immediately put the corpses up for dissection indicated he thought he had nothing to hide, and had no suspicion of the atrocious means by which they had been produced. However, the committee did feel he had acted *incautiously* in believing that poor people of the lowest classes were so ready to sell the bodies of their relatives who had died. The committee believed that Knox had accepted this when Burke and Hare had put it up as the reason why they had so many fresh corpses to offer. They also thought he had been unwise, even though he was a busy man, to leave so much of the purchasing of bodies to his assistants, instead of scrutinizing the purveyors himself.

People saw it as a white-wash report and still clamoured for

Knox's arrest. But was he guilty of criminal knowledge? It is difficult to say with any certainty. He was arrogant and had the callousness of his class and profession of those times. We wouldn't see such indifference again until the arrival of Hitler, Himmler and the concentration camps, in which several hundred doctors abused their training by carrying out experiments on prisoners who hadn't volunteered to be guinea pigs.

But Knox certainly wasn't in this class. He had only experimented upon and dissected the dead. The clearest and best judgement on the doctor and the controversy was probably that from his eminent contemporary, Professor Robert Christison, the professor of Medical Jurisprudence at Edinburgh University. He described him as "a man of undoubted talent, but one who is notoriously deficient in principle and in heart. He was exactly the sort of person who would blind himself against suspicion and fall into a blame-able carelessness." He added however, "But it is absurd to charge him with anything else."

And this, I think, would be about right. It wasn't only a matter of personal and professional pride but also rivalry. Knox wanted more bodies than his competitors were getting, and if they were fresh, so much the better. It was economics too, for more students meant a better income. There were many reasons therefore, why Knox was willing to beguile himself into believing that the poor in the slums were always willing to sell their dead relatives, and if the dead were slow in dying and were given a nudge on the way, well he, Knox, hadn't actually seen it happen. As, when a century and a quarter later, Professor Hirt at the anatomical institute of Strasbourg University asked the Gestapo for fresh corpses, he could say that he didn't see how they were actually acquired.

No doubt Knox's sense of class superiority helped his complacency, and when linked with his intellectual arrogance and professional dedication, became a powerful weapon against caring, or even wishing to know, from whence came the *beef*. If he suspected Burke and Hare at all, and I believe he must have guessed the truth, it was only the troublesome poor murdering the troublesome poor. They were of little use alive, he might well have decided, but could be of value in improving scientific knowledge once dead.

Dr Knox's silence didn't save him. It was taken as just another indication of his guilt at worst, his arrogance at best. By the 1830s his name was mud. Few people would send their sons to him for training in anatomy. He decided to leave Edinburgh and tried, unsuccessfully, for appointments at several universities. Later he settled at Hackney, in London, a comparatively poor man by this time. Eventually he was appointed anatomist to the London Cancer Hospital. Meanwhile the government had regularized dissection and care was taken that no body was sent to a dissection establishment who hadn't announced their wishes on this matter before their death.

There was another bloody piece of dissection in Edinburgh. This was of William Burke. Fresh from the gallows he was hurried to a dissecting table – at the express wishes of the sentencing judge. Here his body was hacked to pieces by a leading anatomist before a specially invited audience of distinguished Scots. Meanwhile, lost in London, Dr. Knox was eventually forgotten. He wrote a successful text-book on anatomy and a book on fishing in Scottish rivers. He died in London in 1862 and if forgotten, he wasn't forgiven.

DR. WILLIAM PALMER

When his racehorse, Polestar, was first past the winning post at the Shrewsbury November Handicap in 1855, John Parsons Cook, with a tact which was commendable but wouldn't save his life, turned to his friend, Dr. William Palmer, and consoled him on his frightful betting losses. The sporting doctor had plunged heavily with money he had borrowed on a horse which was still running.

It was a fine day for an English November, with heat still in the sun, and the meeting was well attended because the virtuous Victorians were relaxing to celebrate the good news at last from the Crimea, where the besieged Russian fort of Sebastopol had fallen. But the happy mood only grated on Dr. Palmer's taut nerves. It seemed that Lady Luck and he had become painfully estranged these past months, even though the dandy doctor was invariably a great success with the ladies.

Ruin, disgrace and even transportation to a penal colony faced him for various acts of fraud as he turned, shrugging and smiling from the rail, and complimented Cook on his good fortune. At least one of them – Cook – had been saved from ruin. Cook thanked him for his thanks, told him that all the drinking and dinner would be on him, and avowed that Palmer's luck must surely change.

Palmer said firmly that it would, as he knew it must. He firmly believed that one made one's own luck, and he had devious ways of manipulating and manufacturing luck so there was very little chance left in it.

Palmer was surprisingly cheerful as they moved through the gay crowds to the nearest tavern, and Cook, who must have known of his friend's mountain of debts and that he was on collision course with prison, suspected nothing. Palmer must have decided on the short walk that Cook would have to go; that although Cook had won, he would lose; and although he had lost, he must win. It was simple, so damned simple. He would poison his friend and collect his winnings. Nothing to it really, Dr. Palmer could reflect with all the confidence of one who had already successfully poisoned some thirteen people to death, all bedded and then buried without the merest ground ripple of suspicion.

After one or two practice runs to test his poisons, the country doctor had begun to poison with a gay abandon. Old relatives were removed for a variety of reasons and Palmer's own illegitimate children were poisoned because they gave either pain to his purse or his patience.

All the victims had died swiftly and tidily, without irritating periods of lingering. Of course the reasons for their demise were mysterious but in those days many deaths were baffling and God, moving in mysterious ways, would be invoked and the matter forgotten.

After the truth came out and Dr. Palmer was arrested for murder, of course people became wise after the event. Nearly everybody in the neighbourhood had a story to tell of how the doctor had poisoned somebody and how suspicious they had been at the time.

Old neighbours remembered strange happenings and recalled the last utterances made by the dying. Soon Palmer was being blamed for every death in the county. But some of the gossip had point. One lady came forward and recalled how troubled Palmer's wife had been on her deathbed – as well she might be – and how she had been most concerned about the safety of her son, the only surviving one of her four children. It seemed that Dr. Palmer had killed his own wife and children and that, in her final illness, Mrs. Palmer had guessed the truth.

But the fact that he had been able to do away with so many people without occasioning an outcry is not indicative of Palmer's cleverness so much as the lack of medical knowledge of the times and the high mortality rate, especially among children. As we will see by the manner in which Palmer carried out the murder of Cook and the way in which he acted afterwards, his performance lacked style, conviction and commonsense. Because of his terrible acting and his bad script the tragedy often bordered on farce.

One thing is clear through the mists of hate that clung to the small town of Rugeley, Staffordshire, for decades after Palmer's execution, and that is that William Palmer was popular until he was found out. He was charming, helpful and generous, and even though he wanted to be considered a gentleman, and chose to live at an aristocratic level – which led to his downfall – he never lost the common touch, and got on well with all classes of people. When an impoverished local became ill Dr. Palmer was invariably the first to call with a hamper of food.

Palmer committed his murders at an early age, between his twenty-fifth and thirtieth birthdays, and during this time he blossomed into a polished practitioner with a pleasing smile and manner. There was a dimple in his chin which had deepened with good living and he had grown fleshy and round in the face and body. He was prematurely bald but, as the girls hastened to tell him, this only made him look more distinguished and helped him succeed as a doctor.

If his accumulating debts ever made him look worried, the townsfolk assumed the reason to be that he was worried about his mother who was the town tart and thus always involved in some colourful scandal. People remembered that both sides of Palmer's family tree spouted degenerates and they admired him all the more for being able to stand clear of the family wrecks. It was known that the family fortune was founded on theft, for Palmer's maternal grandfather had decamped with the money and the illegitimate daughter of the wealthy woman he had been living with and had settled in Rugeley.

Their daughter, Sarah, married one of her numerous lovers who owned a local sawmill, and the family fortune continued to grow over the years through the theft of timber from the nearby estate of the Marquis of Anglesea – the same Marquis who had buried his leg under a tree at the Battle of Waterloo.

William's father died and left £75,000 but because the family was large, he received only £9,000 which he wouldn't inherit until he was twenty-one. He had done well at school. He had a fine brain and the only criticism was that he was lazy. Later it would be put around that he cheated at exams, cribbed from better pupils and was a bully to boot.

His mother sent him as an apprentice to Messrs. Evans of Liverpool, who were manufacturing chemists, and there William was introduced to drugs and poisons. He developed a taste for the faster life but because the women were frequently quicker than the horses he backed, William was soon in debt. The solution was simple. He stole money from letters sent to the firm for drugs and then threw the letters away without forwarding the goods.

It was back to his mother for William and she repaid his thefts to save him from prison, and then sent him as a private pupil to a Dr. Edward Tylecote at Haywood, in nearby Cheshire. Dr. Tylecote was soon regretting the day that William came. He became such an ardent chaser of local women and distant race meetings that he was something of a spent force at surgery in the mornings. But Dr. Tylecote was amazingly tolerant, for William spent some four years in his employment. During this time William established something of a local record by fathering fourteen illegitimate children.

It is also claimed that William carried on a private practice as an abortionist. But this seems strange, unless he was inefficient at it, because even his own girl friends had to wait nine months to get rid of their own troubles. What is better substantiated is that at about this time, before he was twenty one, William had committed his first murder. He had left Tylecote and taken a job in Stafford Infirmary. The victim was a farmer named Abbey, who had an attractive wife. Mrs. Abbey could often be seen tripping lightly into the outpatient's room (on those days when William was duty doctor) as if she didn't have an ill in the world.

Rumour said that they were having an affair and one evening, when the Abbeys and William were drinking together, William bet the farmer that he doubted that he could drink two glasses of brandy straight off. Abbey accepted the bet, won it, and died two hours later. There was gossip at the inquest, but nothing tangible against William, although it was suggested years later that William had laced the drink with strychnine. But Palmer's motive for this murder, if it was murder, would seem to be obscure. The affair with Mrs. Abbey, if it had been that strong, had been over for some time, and Abbey certainly bore Palmer no grudge.

Nor did William's friendship with the widow blossom after the husband was out of the way.

Another victim who followed Abbey, it was said, was one of William's own children by a girl named Jane Mumford. She died shortly after William had bounced her on his knee in his surgery. There is no evidence that he killed Mr. Abbey or the child, but although the infant mortality rate was very high in those days, William's bastards seemed to die at a faster rate than average. It was suggested at the time of his trial that he would paint his fingers with a mixture of poison and sugar and let the child lick his fingers while he jollied him or her on his knee.

Although William had such a high number of illegitimate children, it seems not to have injured his professional standing in the community or to have hardly tarnished his good name. The time when William could be ostracized from the middle classes and even ruined for producing quantities of children outside wedlock was a good decade away.

When he was twenty two, his mother decided he should round off his medical education by training at St. Bartholomew's in Smithfield, London, but his teachers there were soon mournfully writing to Mrs. Palmer that his chances of passing the rigid examinations were slender. He had a fine brain, they wrote, but he spent too much of his time roistering about London to be fresh and alert for morning classes.

Mrs. Palmer had William's same determination and she had decided that her son was to be a qualified doctor. She paid a famous medical coach, Dr. Stendhall, to cram William, and he was granted an MRCS (Eng) in 1846, when he was still twenty two. It was in keeping with the spirit of the Palmer family that Dr. Stendall didn't get a hundred guineas of his fee until he took Mrs. Palmer to court.

Just a year later, and with a wife now, William returned to Rugeley, and put up his plate at a house not too far from the sprawling mansion where his mother lived in riotous and scandalous splendour. Everybody took to William's wife. She was sweet yet sad, the daughter of a Colonel Brookes and his housekeeper Mary Thornton. The Colonel, said to be an eccentric, refused to marry Mary Thornton even after their daughter was born, and she became so violently bad tempered because of this that the Colonel, who had faced his country's enemies stoically, committed suicide rather than face her daily tirade. There was a botch up in the will and lawyers drained off most of the old soldier's money, but the daughter, Anne, a Ward of Chancery, brought £8,000 with her when she married William.

William met Anne through Dr. Tylecote and one of her guardian's, a Dr. Knight, and both these men were against the marriage because of William's notorious reputation. But Anne loved William and she saw it as a golden opportunity for him to settle down with a medical practice and live down his reckless past.

William, who seems to have been incapable of loving anybody, certainly not his own children and certainly not the gentle Anne, saw the sovereigns of his wife's inheritance as eight thousand golden opportunities. He wasn't one to let other openings go by the board either, for within the year one of the housemaids was big with William's child. William soon had a healthy practice, even if his patients, because of his indifferent and lackadaisical manner, remained unhealthy. He was a member of a large local family and they felt duty-bound to bring their ailments to him.

William was aided, too, by the fact that his only competition at this time was a Dr. Bamford, who was in his eightieth year. Dr. Bamford had practised all his life in Rugeley, was respected and admired, but was uneven in his step and faulty in his focus. Although he was by now incapable of any serious medical duties, William would shortly find work for Dr. Bamford to do – signing death certificates.

Anne Palmer, pregnant herself by now, was forgiving in the

matter of the pregnant housemaid and she suggested that the child be put out with a fosterparent so the maid could continue with her work. William was hesitant because of the fee, but eventually gave in. Sometime later the child was brought to him in the surgery, at his request, so that he might see how it progressed. Just a few hours after this visit the child died in painful convulsions.

William, having wasted his own £9,000, soon got through Anne's inheritance, and since his mother wouldn't lend him any more money, he turned to his mother-in-law, Mary Thornton. The bad-tempered Mary didn't like William but gave him money to stop him being beastly to Anne. Soon William suggested that Mary Thornton come and live with them, and this she did three years after the marriage.

She was not long in the house, however, before she crumbled with severe stomach pains and William called in Dr. Bamford for a second opinion. The octogenarian, who was allergic to controversy, it seems, confirmed William's own theory that it was a bilious condition and he recommended that she be given effervescing mixtures and William suggested he write a prescription for these. In the week that Mary Thornton had left, the St. Bart's graduate fought manfully to save her, fetching and carrying, and not only suggesting medicines and foods but preparing them, and carrying them to her himself.

Dr. Bamford suggested that Dr. Knight be called for Mary was his patient, but this was the same Dr. Knight who had been against Anne's marriage and who didn't like William. When Dr. Knight asked William at the funeral why he hadn't been sent for, which was his right both as doctor and friend, William blandly said that Mary Thornton hadn't wanted him.

Just before she died, Mary Thornton roused herself and, pointing at William, screamed, "Take that devil away." But nobody at the time read any significance into this. William had Dr. Bamford sign the death certificate. He had him do this with all his victims, managing to create the impression, with a nod and a wink, that it gave the old man something to do and made him feel still important.

Although Mary Thornton left £12,000, it was in trust and Anne could only get the interest – and William was facing an army of pressing creditors. He had already been barred from Tattersalls and the better type of sportsmen refused to trade with him. He owed a brewer, Leonard Bladon, £600. Bladon had the misfortune to win £500 at the Chester races and to collect the bet in cash on a day that he had William with him. The success cost him his life. William suggested he come home with him so that he could collect what he owed him. Bladon, delighted the debt was to be paid, agreed, but dropped a note off to his wife, without William's knowledge, to tell her of his good fortune.

Bladon also visited his brother, a shoemaker, in the neighbourhood, told him of his good luck and on the strength of it ordered an expensive pair of boots to be made. He was happy and healthy when he left for Palmer's house but no sooner was he in the drawing room than he was mysteriously struck down.

William soon had Bladon abed and was huffing and puffing about him and telling him that nothing much was wrong. A bad attack of indigestion, he suggested, and he would soon put him right. Bladon was crippled in the same way, the servants noticed, as Mary Thornton had been a few months before. A friend of Bladon's, who chanced by, asked William if Mrs. Bladon had been informed, but William said that Bladon would soon be up and about. There was no need to alarm that good lady, he maintained.

William took the precaution of getting a second opinion and Dr. Bamford eventually arrived. William told him what he thought was wrong and the old man, after a careful examination, agreed. A day later Bladon's friend looked in, thought Bladon looked worse and, horrified that his wife hadn't been informed, left to fetch her.

When Mrs. Bladon reached Rugeley it was but one step ahead of the Reaper. "I was about to send for you, ma'am," William told her at the front door. "I fear your husband has taken a turn for the worse." Bladon, now unconscious, was dead within the hour.

Mrs. Palmer looked after the swooning Mrs. Bladon while Dr. Bamford signed the death certificate and the undertaker, at William's call, walked a familiar path to the Palmer home. Mrs. Bladon became suspicious when she discovered no money, not even a copper coin, in her husband's clothes. But before she could summon the nerve to mention this to William, he brought up the matter of money himself.

Blandly apologizing for mentioning money at such a tragic moment, but excusing his conduct by adding that he had several outstanding debts, William told her that Leonard Bladon owed him sixty pounds. Mrs. Bladon was dumbfounded. After all, she had received a letter from her husband saying not only that he had won £500 but that he was collecting a further debt from William.

She discussed the matter with friends and relatives, including the shoemaker brother, and all advised her to go to the authorities. But she demurred at this. She had stayed as a guest in

Palmer's house, liked him, and could not think anything ill of him. And perhaps, who knows, her husband might have had a boastful streak. Shortly after this another of William's creditors, named Blyth, died. When the widow called on William for the £800 her husband had told her on his deathbed that William owed him, William gave his soft sigh and claimed Blyth had been delirious and the widow had got the story the wrong way round. Actually it was Blyth who owed him £800 but, gallantly, William didn't press for payment.

William had decided that children were an unnecessary expense and only his eldest son, William, who was born in 1848, survived into manhood. Four children born at a yearly rate between 1850 and 1854, died in infancy after, it was said, being bounced on papa's knee in his surgery.

Although we cannot be sure of his motive, William next began to strike down some of his elderly relatives. The first to go was colourful "Beau" Bentley, an uncle much given to heavy drinking. Like the late farmer Mr. Abbey, William challenged "Beau" that he couldn't sink two glasses of brandy straight off. "Beau" did, but died three days later. Next he tried to remove an aunt who was invited to stay. But she decided not to take some pills he insisted she swallow for her health sake. Not wishing to offend him, she tossed them from a bedroom window. Next morning she noticed that several of the Palmer's chickens were dead, but she saw no significant link with the jettisoned pills until much later.

Much of William's precarious financial position was caused by the fact that he had established his own racing stable in 1852. This involved him in the purchase of buildings, pasture, and in the employment of a jockey and a groom. The biggest expense of all, of course, was the buying of horses. His extravagance and his cavalier attitude to his practice annoyed his neighbours and lost him patients. A year later he was firmly in the grip of moneylenders and, because of the exorbitant interest rates, ended up more in debt than ever.

In an attempt to recoup, he blithely forged his mother's signature to securities, borrowed more money and began to back outsiders heavily. All he needed was a couple of twenty-to-one winners to become solvent again. So that his mother wouldn't receive any correspondence about his forgeries, William had the Rugeley postmaster, Sam Cheshire, first bring him all letters arriving for his mother – an act which later got Sam a term of imprisonment.

About this time, too, William thought of the life insurance angle. He seems to have been the first murdering doctor to think of this idea, which has been copied by so many murderers since. In Rugeley lived a solicitor named Jeremiah Smith who was agent for the Prince of Wales Insurance Company. William took out a life cover for his wife Anne for £13,000. Although she was still a healthy twenty seven years of age, the annual premium was a staggering £750, an amount, understandably, that William had no intention of paying more than once.

When Anne went down with a cold a few months later, William used this as the excuse for giving her a death-dealing complaint. He began dosing her with antimony. Dr. Bamford dutifully answered his call to give a second opinion; confirmed Palmer's findings that Anne had a heavy cold which was aggravated by a run-down condition; and suggested that Dr. Knight, William's enemy and Anne's guardian, also be consulted. Dr. Knight arrived and was of the opinion that Anne was suffering from cholera. He stayed for two days and Anne improved so much under his supervision, that he returned to Stafford.

He got an urgent call to return within three days but Anne was dead on his arrival. All three doctors certified that Anne had died from cholera, and William tearfully recorded in his diary that night:

"Saw the last of my dear wife. Forever. How desolate life is." But William wasn't alone in bed that night. He was comforted by the housemaid who bore him a child nine months later. But next morning, the weeping William told a neighbour: "My poor Anne is dead. I shall not be long here, I fear, before I follow her."

The fact that a healthy young woman had died so soon after being heavily insured made the insurance company suspicious, but they couldn't withhold payment when they saw two independent signatures on the death certificate. William paid off most of his debts with the money, but he still owed £2,000 on a forged bill to a money-lender named Padwick. Padwick was pressing him grimly, which might have added conviction to William's performance at his wife's funeral. Sobbing bitterly, William called to the Heavens: "Take me, God, take me . . . so that I might be with my darling treasure." William had nothing to fear. His turn would come . . . within the year.

Because his stable and racing activities took up most of his time, William took another doctor in to share his practice even though it split the income. William had bounce now. If the bookmakers weren't kind to him, there was always the insurance companies, and he next insured his brother, Walter. Walter had only one ambition in life, it was said, and that was to drink himself to death. William must have reasoned that what was a brother for but to help a brother? The seemingly unsuspecting solicitor, Jeremiah Smith, was asked to arrange a stupendous £82,000 life cover on Walter and, at first, the Prince of Wales Company was not approached. Two other companies, however, turned down the offer after checking and discovering that Walter was an alcoholic.

Finally, to William's surprise, it was the Prince of Wales Company, which, without a query, covered Walter's life for £14,000. William next got Walter lodgings in a hotel in the centre of the town and hired a drunken couple to look after him. William's only instruction to them was to ensure that Walter had fresh bottles of brandy and gin by his bed when he awoke in the morning. They were told to go careful on the food because Walter had a weak stomach and too much food was bad for him. Soon Walter was writing happily to his estranged wife, Agnes, that "William is so kind" and "Now drink is always at my elbow."

William was a daily visitor. It was almost as if Walter was a patient. He would eye any bottle which was too full and chidingly joke, "You can drink faster than that, Walter." But six months passed and Walter's constitution seemed to be standing up to the assault. Another premium would shortly be due, so, perhaps reluctantly – Walter was his brother after all – he gave him a shove with prussic acid pills. Walter died just two evenings after William administered them, and William, with his usual efficient and bustling haste, had Walter buried before his estranged wife, Agnes, even heard of it. She arrived, post-haste, and told William that she was annoyed with him on several counts. First, she hadn't been informed that Walter was ill. Secondly, she hadn't known that William had insured his brother. She was especially incensed because William's first words to her was that Walter owed him money which, he had said, Agnes would pay. Agnes not only refused to pay William, but the insurance company refused also.

William, without waiting for the second policy to pay off, looked around for other subjects, and his stable boy, George Bates (who was regarded locally as the village idiot), was proposed for a life cover of £25,000. He was described for the purpose as "a gentleman of leisure and a landowner with substantial holdings."

Insurance detectives arrived from London, however, and found landowner Bates digging up turnips on a patch of ground behind his hovel. He eagerly admitted that he had signed the form at his employer's request on the understanding that he would get a thousand pounds. Bates said also that his income was rather less than a £1 a week. The detectives next called on William. They told him they suspected that Walter, and Mrs. Palmer, had been poisoned and said the matter would be investigated. William told them that he rather doubted that there was a murderer in the district but agreed that it "was right and proper" things be checked.

A money-lender named Pratt, who had also help arrange the insurances, now pressed for payment of notes William had forged in his mother's name, and it was with this threat of exposure and imprisonment hanging over him that William went to the races in November with John Cook. Just prior to their leaving for the racecourse at Shrewsbury, William heard that the bellhop at the hotel where Walter had died had been talking to the two detectives. Apparently the boy, named Myatt, had told the men that he had seen William put something in Walter's drink just before he died. William not only had a pleasant chat with Myatt, but treating the servant suddenly as an equal, invited him to drink with him. After several drinks with the doctor in the better end of town Myatt went down with a severe stomach complaint, and his ultimate recovery was possibly due to the fact that William was at the Shrewsbury races. When Polestar won, it was champagne and steaks on a jubiliant John Cook at *The Raven Inn*. He had collected £700 in cash and another £1,200 waited him at Tattersalls in London. Shortly after dinner, Cook was taken ill and a local doctor gave him a light emetic. Cook said, "I think I've been poisoned by Billy." But William, laughing, told him he had drunk too much. Cook also told another friend that he thought Palmer had dosed his drink but it is hard to decide whether or not this was jesting. It is possible that since Palmer was a doctor and there had been a number of tragedies about him recently, his acquaintances had adopted the habit of joking about poisoning among themselves. Certainly, throughout his final illness, Cook allowed Palmer to help him. But Palmer sought out the friend the next morning and denied tampering with Cook's drink. "He was damned drunk, that's all. I never play such tricks."

William's horse, The Chicken, was running this day and they went to watch it. William backed it with every penny he could muster. The Chicken lost, which was a tragedy for Cook, for it cooked his goose for him. Cook accompanied Palmer to Rugeley and put up at *The Talbot Arms*, which was opposite William's home. Cook dined with him that night and servants would testify that Cook wasn't drunk when he returned to the inn. Palmer was at the tavern first thing in the morning demanding a pot of coffee to take up to his friends' room. They told him that Cook liked tea in the morning, but Palmer insisted on coffee which is less likely to betray poison.

He gave as reason for his actions that Cook had been drunk the night before. It is almost certain that he placed antimony in the coffee, and this indicated Palmer's technique. He would make the victim sick with antimony which would put him to bed for several days and mystify the medical experts. Then after the victim had been ill for several days, William would administer the *coup de grace*, strychnine, the hard to trace vegetable poison. Naturally, the coffee made Cook violently ill, and Palmer, demonstrating concern and affection, raced between the inn and his house all day. He annoyed the inn's management by sending a girl to another hotel for a bowl of broth. A serving girl who took this up to Cook and tasted it out of curiosity, probably to compare it with their own soup of the day, was sick, as was Cook after drinking it. The faithful Dr. Bamford soon arrived and scolded Cook for drinking too heavily. Cook said he had had but two glasses of wine the night before.

Early next morning Palmer again arrived with coffee, but now he was dressed for town. His creditors were closing in and it forced him to hasten to Tattersalls to collect Cook's £1,200 winnings even before the victim was dead. His time-table was so tight that he raced to London, collected the money, called on several moneylenders, then raced back to Rugeley. With only Dr. Bamford attending him, Cook recovered sufficiently to get up and even get dressed by lunch-time. Palmer had another chore at Rugeley before returning to Cook.

He called on a new doctor in the town, Dr. Charles Newton, and, breathlessly said, "I can't stop . . . it's not a social visit . . . in a hurry . . . lend me three grains of strychnine, please." Dr. Newton immediately complied.

Back at his home, Palmer paused only to inject the drug into pills, hurried across to the hotel and made a much-improved Cook swallow them. Back at his own home, Palmer went to bed fully dressed, it appears, to await the call which he knew would shortly come. The call came. Cook was screaming in torment. But dammit, he didn't die. Palmer sat brooding while Cook tossed and turned in a bad sleep on the bed. He puzzled a maid by making some slanderous remarks about Dr. Newton; puzzled because she knew that only Palmer and Bamford were caring for Cook. When Bamford arrived in the morning, Palmer, who was creating the atmosphere throughout that Cook was Bamford's patient, told the old man that Cook had been taken bad in the night but hadn't wanted him disturbed.

Leaving Cook in Bamford's charge, Palmer tilted off at full speed to get more death-dealing drugs. What if Cook recovered and went to Tattersalls for his winnings? He went to a certain chemist in the town for the first time in two years as bad feeling existed between him and the owner. He ordered prussic acid. While he was waiting in the shop he saw Dr. Newton approach and rushed to block him in the doorway before he could come in. Palmer whispered to Newton that he had something of a confidential matter to discuss and led him to a deserted patch of pavement.

Palmer only made meaningless small talk while he waited for his package, but successfully blocked the doorway to Newton so the doctor didn't know what he was ordering. Next Palmer sent a note to his obliging postmaster friend, Sam Cheshire, asking him to lend him a receipt stamp. Sam Cheshire brought it round himself but was horrified to discover that Palmer wanted it to stamp a cheque for £350 made out supposedly by Cook to Palmer. Palmer said Cook had been too ill to write the cheque himself.

The cheque had disappeared by the time Palmer stood trial but had he been able to prove that it was genuine, it would have gone a considerable way to establishing his defence that he and Cook betted in a partnership and that a substantial part of Cook's winnings on Polestar were his own. Cook's own doctor, William Jones, rushed over from Shrewsbury after receiving a letter from Palmer to say his patient was undergoing a bad bilious attack. "The first thing I noticed," Dr. Jones said later, "was that whatever Mr. Cook was suffering from it wasn't bilious."

Palmer returned with a box of pills while Jones was still there and made a great point of showing him the lid of the box, saying, "Don't you think Dr. Bamford's handwriting is vigorous for a man of eighty?"

Then Palmer, after seeing these pills given to Cook, returned to his own home. He didn't have long to wait. The call that Cook was dying came at midnight, and Palmer was up, dressed and across the road in three minutes. "I never dressed so quickly in my life," he later volunteered.

Cook died in a final convulsion of agony so fierce that it left his body bent backward like a bowstring with his head almost reaching his feet. Dr. Jones, an experienced medical practitioner, was so overcome that he rushed from the room. Later, Palmer gave him £5 and a gold watch, "All the poor beggar had left," he said. Palmer hurried to see Sam Cheshire, the post master, and asked him to witness a document which showed Cook owed him £4,000. Sam refused. Next Palmer shot off to see his old friend, the undertaker, in order to rush the burial. If people were suspicious, they were only vaguely so. Something was wrong obviously, but such was Palmer's bubbling charm and personality that nobody, while in his presence, could think ill of him. Cook's death was mysteriously strange but so were many deaths.

Palmer would have got away with this murder as well but for one Mr. William Stevens. If Palmer was a bit of a busybody, Stevens was more so. He was obstinate, irritable and prejudiced and he didn't like Palmer "the moment I clapped eyes on the fellow." Mr. Stevens was also Cook's stepfather and had been sent for by Dr. Jones. He objected to his stepson's gambling and nefarious friends. But there were other reasons for disliking Palmer. The doctor had interfered by arranging the burial before he arrived. Cook, Stevens said, would be buried in his mother's grave in London. Palmer also annoyed Mr. Stevens by saying almost immediately that Cook owed him £4,000 and by frequently referring to his stepson (in conversation) as that "poor deceased beggar."

Stevens must have decided that Palmer lacked a certain sensitivity (considering he had claimed to be his friend), to repeatedly harp on the fact that Cook had died penniless. At one stage Stevens asked Dr. Jones to fetch down his stepson's betting book, but Jones returned and said he couldn't find it. Stevens was surprised. He knew that Cook methodically listed all his bets mentioning what he owed and what was owed to him. Palmer interjected, "It's not important. It's of no use to find it." Stevens replied sharply, "I'll be the judge of that."

Palmer, persisting, added, "I assure you it is of no use. When a man dies, his bets are done with." He maintained that Cook had done all his betting in cash on the course. But Stevens answered, just as firmly, that he knew what his stepson did and he had heard talk that his stepson had done well at Shrewsbury.

Later he brought up the matter of an autopsy. He wanted to find out what had caused the death; but Dr. Bamford and Dr. Jones were generally against it. During this debate the usually chatty Palmer stood back disinterestedly as if this was a medical matter and therefore out of his province.

Before he left for London, Stevens asked that his stepson's room be locked. His solicitor in London suggested he take his suspicions to a lawyer in Rugeley and recommended one for the purpose. The London station was crowded but who should Stevens spot there as he was on his way back to Rugeley but Dr. Palmer. How odd. It almost seemed as if he was following him about. Mr. Stevens told Palmer on the journey that he would demand a post mortem, and Palmer, apparently without concern answered, "No trouble. That will be easy to arrange."

Farce which was never far from the surface in Palmer's short career now showed itself in the way he dogged Stevens' footsteps. Palmer would pop up at his elbow all over the town as Stevens worked energetically and bombastically to get an investigation going. Palmer insisted on forcing himself on Stevens company at dinner in *The Talbot Arms* in the evenings and Stevens kept the bad news coming. "I think it right to warn you, sir," he said, "that I have had a rather different account of Mr. Cook's affairs today. It appears that he won a considerable amount on Polestar."

Palmer only showed mild interest. "It can all be settled pleasantly," he replied.

Stevens, as if recalling the "deceased beggar" taunts, snapped, "Sir, it will be settled in the courts."

Palmer knew that Stevens was arranging an autopsy and went to see Dr. Bamford, expressing mild surprise that the old fellow hadn't issued a death certificate for Cook. But Dr. Bamford said, "I thought he was your patient so I was leaving the matter to you." Palmer said he thought Bamford, as the senior doctor during the illness, should issue it. Dr. Bamford ascribing death due to apoplexy.

Stevens had got people in sleepy Rugeley talking and if Palmer was aware of the ground swell of gossip about him, he sailed through it imperviously. If anything, during this period when both the law and his creditors were swooping in, he was more the life and soul of the neighbourhood than ever. He kept close to Stevens who was the most dangerous of his opponents.

It is not difficult to imagine those evenings in the bright tap-room and dining room of *The Talbot Arms*, with Stevens rolling off the snide accusations and sarcasms and with Palmer grinning his way through them like a sleek frigate through a storm. No matter how offensive Stevens became, he couldn't drive Palmer away. And Palmer had other troubles at this time as a money-lender's writ had been laid against him which would mean he would be exposed for fraud.

On the Sunday evening when Palmer, with his usual grin in place, bounced into the bar, Stevens asked him if he had been his son's doctor during his final illness. Palmer said he hadn't been, but wanted to know why he asked. Stevens answered. "My son is to be opened up the morning and if you were his doctor it is only fair you should be there."

Perhaps the more farcical incidents in Palmer's career began now as he tracked down the two doctors brought in for the autopsy. To Dr. Harland he said, "I'm glad you are to come to make the post mortem. Somebody might have been sent that I didn't know." When Harland said that there were rumours that Cook had been poisoned, Palmer replied, "I wasn't the doctor but Cook was my friend so I was close, and, poison, I think not. Oh, no. He had an epileptic fit on Monday and Tuesday, and you will find old diseases in the heart and the head." Palmer added with a chuckle, after ordering fresh drinks, "Be on your guard, my friend. There is a very queer old man beating the matter up. He suspects me of something and appears to imagine that I have got the betting book. But Cook had no betting book which could be of any use to anyone."

Palmer not only invited himself to the autopsy, but tried to get Dr. Charles Newton, who was also participating, drunk before he got there. Insisting there was time for a drink, he gave him a tumbler of brandy, saying sympathetically: "You'll need this. It's going to be a dirty job. You'll find that this fellow was riddled with diseases. He had a diseased throat. He had syphilis, and he took a great deal of mercury."

The room where the post mortem was carried out was small and Palmer treated the affair as a joke. Harland had only one jar to contain the organs which would be sent to London for tests. Besides Harland, there was Doctors Newton, Jones and Bamford standing against the table and in the rear, making tart remarks, stood Palmer. Cook's stomach was opened so that the contents could be poured into the jar. As this was in progress, Newton suddenly lunged against Harland, the liquids missed the jar and spilt to the floor. It transpired that Palmer had given Newton a sudden push so he would cannon into Harland at that delicate moment. Palmer also looked behind him to suggest that somebody had come in and pushed him. He also looked at the ancient Dr. Bamford, as if to blame him. Later, laughing, he nudged Bamford and said, "They won't hang us yet."

He kept up a mood of hilarity throughout, striving to convince everybody that Stevens was an old fool and a damned busybody, and that he had no right to question the findings of the eminently respected Dr. Bamford.

A little of Cook's stomach contents got into the jar but Palmer was taking no chances and he attempted to bribe the boy who was carrying the jar to the train by pony and trap to have an accident so that the cart overturned. There were more delays while Guy's Hospital in London called for further organs, as those that had been supplied were not sufficient for the tests. Back in Rugeley, Palmer was active. He was encouraging a friendship with the County Coroner by sending him game he claimed he had just recently killed. If the Coroner was suspicious by the sudden show of friendship by Palmer, he kept it to himself.

Palmer was the first to know of any news from Guy's Hospital, for Sam Cheshire obligingly opened any letters from there and showed them to him before sending them to the authorities. Eventually Guy's came up with the news that they couldn't find any strychnine in Cook's remains. Palmer not only got the information in Rugeley before anybody else, but let the Coroner know in a note he sent him with more game. The authorities conferred. It was agreed that Palmer's actions were peculiar and that there was a great deal of suspicious evidence against him which, if processed in court, might build into a sound circumstantial case against him. The Coroner's court sat and brought in a verdict of wilful murder against the doctor. More evidence was found against him after his arrest for the bodies of his wife and brother were exhumed, and traces of antimony were found in their remains.

So intense was local feeling against Palmer that it was decided that if he were to have a fair trial it would have to be carried out elsewhere. A special law, still known as the Palmer Act, was rushed through parliament. This empowered a prisoner to elect for trial in London if he thought he wouldn't get a fair hearing in his own district. People knew that many murders in the past had been carried out by poison, but poisoners, until just recently, had rarely been caught. The science of toxicology was but still a weak infant, and Palmer's trial, for this reason as much as the hilarity of it all, caused international interest.

He stood trial at the Old Bailey in May 1856 ten years (almost to the day) after he had graduated from nearby Bart's Hospital. The prosecution was led by the Attorney-General, as is usual in poison trials. This man, Sir Alexander Cockburn, handled the case so skilfully, that even Palmer, who suffered by it, was full of admiration for him. After he was sentenced to death, William turned to his solicitor and said, "Cockburn's great riding did it for me."

Palmer was executed publicly in Stafford. The gallows were built high so that the huge crowd, that was expected, could see him. He came through the gates of the prison smiling. He moved with his usual fast and nervous bounce, suggesting as always that he was an important man in a great hurry on essential business. He died with his smile still in place.

For a time Rugeley was a hotbed of interest. Everybody had a Palmer story, and people claimed they had been made ill just by speaking to him, let alone drinking with him or swallowing his pills. But soon Rugeley wanted to forget Palmer and they asked for government permission to change the name of the town. It brought a memorable pun from the Prime Minister, Lord Palmerston: "Certainly they can change it," he said, "why don't they name it after me?"

Only one person wept at the time; Palmer's mother. She overlooked the fact that William had killed another of her sons, the drunkard Walter, and many of her grandchildren, and observed that she had had seven children but that William was the best and kindest of the lot. Breaking down, she screamed, "They've hanged my saintly Billy."

DR. THOMAS SMETHURST

Although William Palmer had been tried and hanged, medical jurisprudence had got off to a shaky start in England. Harried by doctors for the defence, the prosecution hadn't established that Palmer's victim, Cook, had died from strychnine poisoning. Even though the public was willing to agree that Palmer was the sort who would kill a creditor if he couldn't make a killing at the racetrack, there was an outcry after his trial because the prosecution hadn't successfully made out its case. However, the public's disquiet was anaesthetized by fact that there were two other murder charges pending against Palmer. What emerged from the trial, and what we still see in similar trials today, was contradictory medical evidence; the prosecution's doctors saying one thing, the defence's pet doctors the opposite. So, as with later juries, this one ignored both sets of medical experts, and found Palmer guilty due to the fact that he had been proved to have purchased poison and had started spending the victim's money before he was dead. But so contradictory and baffling was the medical testimony at the trial that the Attorney-General, in his final address to the jury, declared:

> "To me, it seems a scandal upon a learned, a distinguished, and a liberal profession, that men should come forward and put forward such speculations as these, perverting the facts, and drawing from them sophisticated and unwarranted conclusions with the view of deceiving the jury."

Perhaps he was being a bit hard on the medical profession, which has never professed to be an exact science, especially when this was coming from a barrister who had mastered the art of twisting-words so successfully that he was the leading lawyer in his profession; a profession which can vehemently demand the death sentence for a villain he is prosecuting one day and freedom if he is defending him the next. But the attorney-general's remarks, unfortunately, are as relevant today as when he made them over a hundred years ago. Juries, composed of laymen, are still asked to adjudicate on contrasting and opposing medical evidence. Dr.

Castaing's trial in France and more especially Dr. Palmer's in London, alerted the potential poisoner to the need to proceed with caution. And with the trial of Dr. Thomas Smethurst, which came just three years after Palmer's execution, there was to be a green light ahead for those who killed by poison. Medical jurisprudence emerged so battered from the Smethurst trial that judges and juries ever since have tended to look for other than medical evidence to indicate guilt or innocence in the defendent.

Like Palmer, Thomas Smethurst was a bit of a bad 'un, but there was nothing you could ever put your stethoscope on and say "Ah" about. There was that little business back in 1826 when he was arrested for buying goods for which he couldn't pay, and that was the same year he married Miss Mary Durham at St. Mark's Church, Kennington. If there was a crime in that, it was Miss Durham's, for she was forty-nine and young Thomas twenty-three, so it was almost a case of kidnapping.

Like so many of the doctors in this work, Smethurst hasn't much to recommend him. He was short and insignificant. After receiving a rather doubtful degree from the University of Erlangen, he practised in London for nine years and then at Ramsgate, Kent, for another three. He also went abroad, presumably on his wife's money, and after studying hydropathy, returned to England and set up a water-cure establishment near Farnham, and there produced a little textbook called *Hydrotherapia*. He thereupon retired when he was forty-eight and we find him, when our story opens, living with his wife in a modest boarding house in the Bayswater Road, London. And it was to this house that Miss Isabella Bankes came in 1858. She was said to be attractive, charming, and a spinster. She was forty-two years old, had a life interest in £5,000 a year which gave her £220 per annum, and had a cachet of capital totalling some £1,800.

The best and most graphic testimony of what happened next came at the trial from the landlady, Mrs. Smith. She had liked Miss Bankes but reported that her digestion wasn't as powerful as it might be for she was subject to bilious attacks. These often sent the lady hastening with embarrassment from her table at meal-times. Perhaps it was this condition which attracted the doctor, who sat with his distinguished and elderly wife on the opposite side of the room. The illness could not have been caused by the toughness of the food for nobody else went down, and the doctor called on the distressed lady offering his services.

But soon the doctor was offering Miss Bankes such private and privileged services that Mrs. Smith put her foot down. She would have none of that in her boarding house and poor Miss Bankes, weak stomach and all, was sent out into the cold. Dr.

Smethurst behaved like a gentleman and offered her his protection. They settled down together in a boarding house at Richmond, after stopping at a church in Battersea for a bigamous marriage.

Smethurst detractors have suggested that the doctor kept from Miss Bankes the fact that he was married to the elderly lady in Bayswater Road and that she consequently didn't know it was a bigamous marriage. It has been suggested that she was told that the woman was an older sister or even his mother. This view would hold more validity if the second Mrs. Smethurst hadn't signed her will *Isabella Bankes* when she executed it just before her death.

Miss Bankes might have been lonely and so much in need of love that her judgement was affected, but it is hard to believe that Smethurst could have given her sufficient reason as to why she should sign her will with her maiden name if she knew she was *legally* married. Why did the doctor commit the then heinous crime of bigamy? Respectability was everything; it didn't matter if it was only a pose. Moreover, it seemed that Smethurst thought that his wife, now 74, would soon die. It was also his way of showing Isabella that his intentions were honourable. He was risking criminal charges for her and demonstrating that a half loaf was better than none. He had docked his age by several years to prove to her that his first marriage had been more a case of child-napping than it actually was and later he would say he committed bigamy for reasons of snobbery. "Miss Bankes was a person of good family and the marriage was a preliminary to another at a future period, and in order that she should be protected from reproach hereafter."

There it was then. Manfully, Smethurst was taking the sin on his own narrow shoulders, even though Isabella definitely knew about his relationship with the old gal in Bayswater. The attitudes of respectable landladies must also have influenced their decision to commit bigamy. They were, after all, fleeing one *respectable* boarding house for another *respectable* boarding house, and they were, especially Miss Bankes, the sort of gentlefolk who could only frequent these types of establishments. A half lie was better than a whole lie then, especially if a strict landlady asked for proof of their marriage. The most important thing was acceptability. People actually murdered rather than be exposed as *not respectable* – and if you disbelieve this, study the motives of several of the murders in this book. This was the 1850s and Victorian virtue was as rampant as the English lion. We shouldn't judge all Victorians, of course, by the Smethursts.

We don't know what the real Mrs. Smethurst thought about

her husband's behaviour. Evidence suggests that she was well into senile decay, and she never pronounced on his actions even if she knew about them. This wife, who was old enough to be his mother, kept quiet on the matter even after his arrest and trial. But Dr. Smethurst kept in touch with her. We know that they corresponded even if the forbidding exterior of Landlady Smith kept him from visiting her. He reassured her, by letter, that he would soon be back with her and Mrs. Smith in Bayswater. This letter was produced at his trial to attempt to show that he was anxious to destroy Miss Bankes in order to return to the frosty welcome of his old landlady.

The newly-weds had only been under the watchful eye of their new landlady, Miss Robinson, for three months, when Isabella fell ill. It was her faulty digestion again. Dr. Smethurst administered to her for a time. Finally, not satisfied with his own work and her lack of progress, he took the landlady's suggestion and called in a local G.P. named Dr. Julius. He also was troubled by the lady's decline and consulted another doctor named Bird. Julius arrived on April 3. By May 3, Isabella was dead.

Before she died, however, several peculiar things had happened. On the Saturday before her death, April 30, Smethurst called on a solicitor named Mr. Senior. He had with him Isabella's will, written in his own hand, and asked Mr. Senior to come round on the Sunday and execute it. Mr. Senior was shocked – or claimed at the trial to be shocked. What, work on the Sabbath? The joyless English Sunday, still with us, was in the ascendant. But Senior, obviously a hypocrite, went presumably to get the fee, even though he said at Smethurst's trial: "I told him that I didn't like to do business on the Sabbath, and the law didn't like wills being executed on a Sunday."

The lawyer was pressed by Smethurst to execute the will as it was a matter of the greatest urgency. But the fact that Smethurst had made the solicitor work on a Sunday obviously counted against him with the jury. Senior certainly went and witnessed the patient's signature. Yet another respectable professional man was profaning that very same Sabbath because of Smethurst. While he was hurrying to the Richmond solicitor, Dr. Alfred Swaine Taylor, Professor of Chemistry at Guy's Hospital, was testing some of Isabella's waste at the request of Dr. Julius and Dr. Bird, who now suspected poison. Dr. Taylor had protested about doing this work on the Sabbath but Julius and Bird had told him of their suspicions. It was Dr. Taylor who had had the thankless task of analyzing the contents of Cook's stomach, after William Palmer had scattered them over the floor at the autopsy. If he didn't actually shine at the Palmer trial, he would go down with a resounding thud come Smethurst's contest with the law. He would make a mistake in his tests so disastrous that the effects would be felt in medical jurisprudence for a century.

Perhaps because it was Sunday, or perhaps Dr. Taylor didn't give reflective thought to his work as he analyzed one of Isabella's stools, because erroneously he found arsenic there. This information, already suspected by doctors Julius and Bird, was carried to the authorities, and Smethurst was arrested on the Monday. He appeared immediately in a magistrate's court, charged with administering poison to Isabella. And, even stranger, he was permitted bail. He told the magistrate that Isabella was very sick and if he was kept in the cells there would be nobody to nurse her at night. The magistrate, a Victorian gentleman, looked at Dr. Smethurst, apparently also a gentleman, and didn't hesitate. He allowed a man who had been charged with attempted murder to go back and nurse his suspected victim. Dr. Smethurst spent the night alone with Isabella and she died next day.

There was shock and horror at the post mortem inquiry, for it was discovered that not only had Dr. Smethurst married Isabella bigamously but that she had been five to seven weeks pregnant. Surprisingly, after Dr. Taylor's tests, no arsenic was found in any of her organs. Minute amounts of antimony, however, were discovered. Nobody, at the moment, looked too closely at the discrepancy in the medical findings because Smethurst, by his bigamy and because his victim was pregnant, had already been exposed as the blackest of all villains.

Smethurst's trial opened at the Old Bailey in July 1859, and the prosecution set out to prove that he had poisoned Isabella in order to get hold of the £1,800 she had owned and also so as to be able to get back to the ancient Mrs. Smethurst and the foxy landlady in the Bayswater Road. The prosecutor, in his first speech, sought to negate any snags by agreeing that Smethurst knew he wouldn't get the £220 annuity which died with Isabella, but that the lump sum of £1,800 was motive enough. Because of the mauling taken by the medical witnesses in the Palmer trial, the prosecution stepped warily. They claimed only that Isabella had been put down by an irritant metallic poison, without specifying which one. One thing these trials were showing was the growing and insatiable appetite of Victorians for murder. Earlier Britons had accepted murder as an affliction which would always be with us and had evinced only moderate interest in these crimes, but Victorians couldn't get enough of the gory details, and a popular press was developing which would feed their thirst. It was as if their new-found piety was so strict that the very deed of murder shocked and fascinated the Victorians by its outlandishness. The judge at Smethurst's trial was so interested in the case that he had deliberately manipulated his cases so that he could try it. If it didn't arouse as much keeness as the Palmer affair, it could only be that advanced publicity had revealed more about Palmer than Smethurst. Little could be found out about the latter doctor because there was little to know; gay, charming, energetic Palmer had littered a county or two with bodies.

But there is gore and gore. The judge, the Lord Chief Baron Pollock, horrified future legal historians by admonishing the prosecution for describing the findings of the post mortem in too graphic detail. One jury-man was led into the street to recover after hearing these results and the judge said it was unnecessary to upset the jury by telling them things which, in any case, they couldn't understand.

If that was the first bombshell, there were others. Here was Dr. Alfred Taylor, manfully but matter-of-factly, telling the court that he had been wrong, and that what he had thought had been arsenic in the victim's waste, wasn't arsenic at all. There was arsenic, he said, but it had come from the copper gauze with which he had carried out the tests. Having made this startling admission, Taylor would still have it, however, that Miss Bankes had been felled by arsenic. He even had a theory how Smethurst had accomplished this. The doctor had given his victim arsenic, he said, and then cunningly he had eliminated it by the administration of chlorate of potass. This theory would be, rightly, ignored by the judge and the jury, and by the medical profession. Dr. Taylor said antimony had been taken from the body, but this amounted to no more than one-half grain. Inflamation and ulceration in the stomach area, he maintained, could only have been caused by an irritant poison. But he was forced to agree with the defence counsel that, if arsenic had been used to kill, it would be found in many parts of the body. No traces of the poison, however, were found in Miss Bankes' remains.

Dr. Taylor was of the opinion that Dr. Smethurst had first used his specialized knowledge of poisons to destroy Miss Bankes and next to destroy most of the evidence of these poisons. Altogether, the prosecution marshalled the support of ten medical men who claimed a foreign substance, an irritant, had killed Miss Bankes and who also said that they didn't think she had died from dysentery or any similar disease.

The defence answered with seven equally eminent members of the medical profession who suggested that she had died from acute dysentery, and they also introduced the possibility, for the first time, that the pregnancy might have been the cause of her death, or at least have speeded it. Defence doctors also claimed that an analysis of grey powder and bismuth – two of the medicines administered to the deceased – carried amounts of arsenic and antimony. Pregnant women, it was said, were liable to dysentery, and heartburn was also a common disorder in this condition; and so, of course, could be vomiting and diarrhoea. Since Miss Bankes wasn't found to be pregnant until after her death, it seemed that neither Dr. Smethurst nor doctors Julius and Bird had either thought it could be a factor in her death or even tested her for this eventuality.

Even though the defence handled itself in a brilliant manner and the evidence of Smethurst's innocence, on the basis of what went on at the trial, is obvious to modern eyes on rereading the case, Smethurst was doomed. He was seen by his contemporaries as a black scoundrel. He had forsaken an old wife after years of her life and much of her money; he had seduced poor Miss Bankes by all sorts of foreign trickery, it was said, and then insulted both church and state by criminally marrying her. Not smitten down with remorse after these deeds, he had made two professional men profane the Sabbath. And it was Smethurst's fault, not Dr. Taylor's, that a mistake had been made on that shattered Sunday. Everybody assumed, trial or no trial, that Smethurst had murdered poor Miss Bankes, mainly because it was in keeping with all that had gone before. His character was obviously counting against him not only with the jury but also with the judge, who should have known better.

Desperately the defence claimed that the prosecution hadn't proved that Miss Bankes had died from poisoning; nor had it proved that Smethurst had even had such poison or had in fact administered it. The prosecution hadn't even proved that the doctor had at all times tried to keep Isabella under his care and control. It had been Smethurst himself who had asked Dr. Julius to give a second opinion and Bird a third. Moreover, he had left the house for visits to London and Richmond on several occasions, leaving Isabella in the care of others. While he had often prepared her food himself, there were many occasions when he had left this chore to others. This point the defence did establish.

The defence also did much to smash the supposed motive for the murder. Dr. Smethurst, it was pointed out, already had sufficient means. Apart from this, Isabella Bankes considered herself his wife, and therefore he had benefit of not only the £1,800 she had in the bank already but the £220 a year which would die with her. Even the small amount of antimony in the deceased's body, maintained the defence, wasn't sufficient to kill and could have come from imperfections in the many medicines she was being dosed with. The prosecution had stipulated that the only reason that no poison had been found in the doctor's possession was because he had got rid of it. But, declared the defence, Dr. Smethurst had first been arrested on the day before Isabella Bankes died, and then re-arrested on the day of her death, so that he had hardly had the time to dispose of any poisons he might have had in his possession.

The defence reminded the court of the fact (which seemed to be worrying nobody) that had not Dr. Taylor discovered his mistake with the arsenical gauze or, having discovered it, kept the matter to himself, Dr. Smethurst would have been hanged on this evidence alone. But the brilliant defence of Mr. Serjeant Parry was wasted on Baron Pollock and the jury. It was said later, in their defence, that they had had the time to study Smethurst in court and could recognize him by his stance as the villain he was. If nobody in court was satisfied of Smethurst's innocence, nobody outside the court was a hundred per cent certain of his guilt. After Smethurst was found guilty, there was a hubbub, especially from the medical press. To be fair to Baron Pollock, he had implied his own doubt when he sentenced Smethurst. But before this, he addressed the jury for nine hours, in which, it is said, he showed bias against the accused. First, Baron Pollock told the jury they must decide if Miss Bankes met her death by poison. If they thought she had, they must next decide if the accused was responsible for poisoning her. Baron Pollock said, however, that the jury shouldn't overlook the fact that while the annual income of £220 died with Isabella Bankes the immediate possession of £1,800 would come to Smethurst on her death.

It might be considered to the favour of the defendant, said the judge, that no poison was found in his possession on his arrest; but the jury shouldn't overlook the fact that the life of Miss Bankes was drawing to a close and that the accused, a medical man, might have decided that no more of the deadly ingredient was needed. Baron Pollock reminded the jury that Smethurst was alone in the house on the last night of Isabella Bankes's life, having been released on bail so that he might attend to her.

The judge said that while it was true Dr. Taylor had indeed made an error in one instance, this was no reason to reject all his other testimony. Other doctors had come forward to state that the deceased might have died from natural causes, said Baron Pollock, but each of them had refrained from stating that this was actually so. He did remind the jury of the telling defence point that if Miss Bankes had been killed by poisons, these should have been found in her body and, in particular, in her liver.

Baron Pollock said he thought little of the defence suggestion that the jury were being asked to decide which medical evidence of the two opposing groups was correct; death by poison or by natural means. While the medical evidence was important, he said, the jury, in addition, must look at all the factors, and, in particular, at the conduct of the accused and at any motives he might have had for committing the crime with which he was charged. He reminded them that they must be guided by rules of commonsense; the commonsense which operates in the minds of reasonable men. Even if there was no medical evidence before them to evaluate, the jury would still have been called on to decide on the guilt or innocence of the defendant.

Baron Pollock talked for nine hours, but the jury took only forty minutes to find Smethurst guilty of murder. Judges then had more power than they do now, and it was within a judge's prerogative to have imprisonment substituted for execution. However when a judge decided that a convicted man didn't deserve to have his life saved, he would intimate as much when he passed the death sentence. In announcing death by hanging and stipulating a date for the execution, he would indicate to the accused that he had no hope of mercy and that he must prepare himself to leave this world. Baron Pollock, however, in announcing the automatic death sentence on Smethurst, didn't add this final phrase. Since poisoning was considered the worst of all forms of murder, anybody convicted of it couldn't hope to escape the gallows.

But Baron Pollock knew more about Smethurst than the jury had been told. He was, due to this secret knowledge of the man (knowledge which was never publicly disclosed), satisfied of his guilt. Baron Pollock knew however that the case hadn't been sufficiently proven in law. He realized that he would have to request the Government to forgo the full penalty in this case.

As Baron Pollock never revealed any of the secrets he knew about Smethurst, we have no way of knowing how they would affect our modern judgement towards his trial. It might be that he was suspected of other serious crimes like murder – crimes which couldn't legally be proven. But knowing how easy it was to upset these early Victorians, it might be only that they had discovered he was a philanderer. Perhaps he had an addiction for seducing lonely spinsters at the respectable boarding houses he frequented, just so as to break the gloomy monotony of his life. Because he might have played a sort of Russian roulette with his respectability, in both trying to seduce spinsters and at the same time avoid being caught out by his straight-laced landladies, one cannot assume, as some Victorians did, that he would murder anybody.

The jury was convinced of Smethurst's guilt. Baron Pollock was hesitant. But the public at large – especially the intellectuals –

were horrified by the findings. Guilty he might be, but it hadn't been proven. The strongest attack on the verdict came from the medical press, who could call on expert medical knowledge. The *Medical Times and Gazette* summed it up in two short sentences: "Is the prisoner guilty? We believe he is. Was he proved guilty? Certainly not." The journal found that while the balance of *probabilities* was against the doctor, there was a *possibility* that he might be innocent.

While maintaining that Smethurst was a cheat and a scoundrel with whom no decent person could feel any sympathy, the *British Medical Journal* said the doubt of his guilt was too great. Pointing out that ten medical witnesses said that Miss Bankes had died by poisoning, and seven others blamed natural causes, the *Journal* said:

> "Here, at least, is a division of opinion in the skilled evidence which should make us pause. Was it an irritant poison, or an irritable uterus, or the ulcerated bowel of dysentery which did the poor lady to death? We confess that, as far as we can judge, her pregnant condition was quite sufficient to account for the symptoms under which she laboured. There is one very remarkable circumstance which has not, we believe, been noticed, namely, that the commencement of the fatal illness tallies very exactly with the commencement of her pregnancy. It may be urged, however, that these mere simulation of symptoms of poisoning, which arise in some cases of pregnancy, affords no proof whatever that this was not a genuine case of poison."

The *Journal* also said that the fact that no poison had been traced to Smethurst, or had been known to have been purchased by him, raised especial doubts, since this had been the essential proof needed in other poisoning trials before the defendant could be convicted. Here was the leading medical journal in Britain, then, suggesting that nobody should be tried on medical evidence alone.

The qualifications of some of the trial doctors came under critical scrutiny. Dr. Julius, for example, had received his doctor's certificate from the Archbishop of Canterbury, because those were the days when the primate could issue such certificates, a patronage dating from Henry VIII. Dr. Smethurst's degree, which came from the University of Erlangen, was considered by many as suspect, for it was thought the university too casually issued these at the drop of a fee. Dr. Pritchard, whose murdering exploits are also included in this book, also got a degree from the university, and didn't leave Scotland to get it.

The medical profession rounded on Dr. Taylor. The *Dublin Medical Press*, discussing the damage he had done his profession, hoped he would withdraw into the obscurity of private life, and take his favourite arsenical copper gauze with him. But Dr. Taylor was to remain and adjudicate on medical matters at many a trial yet.

The majority of people might consider Smethurst guilty but the point was – and we must admire the Victorians for their stand here – he hadn't been proven so, and the public wouldn't have it. Some sixty doctors and barristers, the leaders in their fields, demanded the release of the prisoner or a re-trial. The government, as governments are wont to do, moved slowly, considered all the facts and later asked a leading surgeon to evaluate the evidence. He did so, confirming the opinion that Smethurst hadn't been proven guilty on the evidence available, and a warrant of pardon was issued.

But Victorians would have their pound of flesh. Smethurst was handed the pardon in one hand and an order for his arrest on a charge of bigamy with the other. He stood trial for this and went to prison for a year. Smethurst had a surprise or two of his own. No sooner was he released than he was bobbing up in court again. Now he was suing the next of kin of Miss Bankes for the £1,800 she had left him under the terms of her will. Smethurst won the case, collected the money, and promptly disappeared – which was wise of him for it was regarded as a dastardly, cheeky act.

Even with more modern techniques, increased knowledge and more sophisticated medical practitioners, we cannot improve enough on the medical findings of the time, as to be able to say now whether Dr. Smethurst was guilty or not. The doctors were pumping half a dozen assorted medicines into Miss Bankes to cure her and this would account for the small amount of antimony found in her remains.

Antimony, a painful and pernicious form of poison, had been made popular by Palmer. Given to a victim over a period of time, as Dr. Pritchard would later do with his wife, it would aggravate any illness or weakness of the victim and would bring about a death which would be assumed to relate to the original disease.

Antimony had lots of uses in Victorian times. Like arsenic, it could be found all over the place. It was often used in stables to give the black coats of the cobs which pulled the coaches a fine gloss. And many a Victorian gentleman, suspecting a servant of taking nips from his decanters, would lace the drink with drops of antimony. The pain which resulted, terribly excruciating, was better than anything else at warning servants off. If Smethurst finished off Miss Bankes with antimony, he must have found a way of draining it from her system, when she was on the point of death.

Nevertheless, the condition of Miss Bankes, after a rereading of the testimony today, shows a death more consistent with an irritant poison. But the fact that she might have died from natural causes, by dysentery aggravated by her pregnancy, cannot entirely be ruled out.

A solution to the mystery, not thought of at the time, is that Dr. Smethurst might have inadvertently brought about Isabella's death by attempting to abort her. This is a fact worth considering because Isabella was fragile and had a weak constitution. She wasn't the doctor's real wife and was, at forty-three, a little too old to have a child with any degree of safety in an age when childbearing was fraught with dangers. It could be that Dr. Smethurst began by doctoring her, with her own knowledge, with daily doses of vegetable, not metallic, irritants, a then popular method of bringing about abortions.

Perhaps this treatment got out of hand. Perhaps Smethurst, aware of the outcome, hurried to get the will executed. Perhaps, however, Isabella had pleaded with him initially to carry through the abortion and, aware that it had gone wrong, insisted that the will be executed so that he, and not her relatives, should have her money. This can only be conjecture. Whatever went on between the charming Isabella and the inscrutable and insignificant doctor can only be guessed at. We will never know. For having collected Isabella's money, the doctor stepped into the obscurity from whence he came and was never heard from again.

DR. EDWARD PRITCHARD

Crime can have produced no greater hypocrite and melodramatic ham actor than the Victorian poisoner Dr. Edward Pritchard. Looking back a century, he seems the epitome of all things we feel reprehensible in Victorian Britain. He used adjectives to a fault in conversation, and ended every sentence he spoke with a theatrical exclamation mark. His religious convictions were transparently insincere and his sentimentality, delivered in grandiloquent rhetoric, bordered on the hysterical.

Thus we see him smiting his forehead and shouting at the body of his dead wife, the woman he had slowly and painfully poisoned over four months, "Come back! Come back my darling Mary Jane! Don't, I beg of you, leave your dear Edward!" Long before the advent of the silent movie in which lack of a sound track called for exaggerated facial contortions and body rackings - Edward Pritchard was a pantomime movie actor.

In a country pre-occupied with religion, Edward Pritchard had shrewdly perceived that the quickest way to popularity was to crash down on your knees at a moment's notice and offer up a prayer. Consequently, it became a habit of his right up to the gallows tree. He was not only one of the greatest and yet most transparent liars that crime has produced – but one of the most vain and conceited. He would carry postcard-sized photos of himself in his pocket and distribute them to anybody he met including even passing strangers on a train. If he could get it, he would charge a fee for these, to help with the printing costs. His statements were outlandish to the point of ridiculousness. He once began a conversation with, "I have plucked the eaglets from their eyries in the deserts of Arabia and I have hunted the Nubian lion in the prairies of North America."

A much less than competent doctor, the only thing Pritchard was said to be good at was humping the more impressible of his women patients over his desk, a habit that got him into trouble. No female was safe, in fact, after the surgery door had clicked closed. He might have had a few successes as he indiscriminately lechered, but he also lost a few patients, and one or two angry husbands came calling. After one such incident he was forced to move. Why Pritchard should murder a mother-in-law he loved and a wife who tolerated his infidelities remains, perhaps, the biggest mystery about him.

Pritchard was born at Southsea, Hampshire, in December of 1825, the son of a naval captain and nephew of a couple of admirals. After some six months at the College of Surgeons, he was gazetted as an assistant surgeon in the Royal Navy, and for the next four years served in the Pacific and the Mediterranean. He was serving in Portsmouth when he met Mary Jane Taylor, who was staying with her uncle, a retired naval surgeon. Mary Jane came from Edinburgh and the suggestion is that she was sent to the naval port to find a husband. She found Pritchard and they married in the autumn of 1850. Naval duties called and the newly-weds were parted, and then it was suggested that the Taylor family buy Pritchard a practice so that they could set up home together.

Pritchard was tall, thickset, good looking and always bent himself to please. He was inordinately proud of his beard which he wore longer than most Victorian gentlemen, and which he spent a good deal of time combing and pomading. Initially his practice, which was at Hunmanby, Yorkshire, prospered. But then there were whispers which, although they didn't become shouts, damaged the practice and would eventually send him fleeing to Scotland. Edward tried to seduce a patient who complained to her husband, and the husband threatened legal action. However, before he could carry this forward, he had died.

By now Pritchard had met defeats on the social front. His colleagues not only avoided conversation with him but would fall silent if his name was introduced into the conversation. The *Sheffield Telegraph* summed up his impact on Hunmanby and Filey by saying, after his arrest: "They found his imagination overran the limits of probability as much as his expenditure overran his means. He left with no credit, only creditors. He was fluent, plausible, amorous, politely impudent and singularly untruthful. The prettiest liar ever met with."

It was said that Pritchard only spoke the truth by accident and only took the back seat at a meeting if all the other chairs were occupied. We don't know what Mrs. Pritchard, or her family, thought of his lack of funds and unpopularity, but by now she had five children to concern herself with. In 1857 Pritchard brought by post a diploma of Doctor of Medicine from the University of Erlangen and became a licentiate of the Society of Apothecaries of London. He was also a member of the Freemasons in Yorkshire but rather annoyed that body by parading about in public in his robes and using the brotherhood to publicize his practice. By 1858, when he was 33, there was nothing to do but get out of Yorkshire before he was kicked out, and after a year spent abroad, he recommenced medical practice in Glasgow in 1860.

Pritchard had only been a short time in Glasgow, practising from 11 Berkeley Terrace, when he again felt the cold finger of ostracization from his colleagues. As usual his patients were vehemently for or against him. He could dash off a prescription with great panache after only a cursory check at the patient while treating him, or more usually her, to a slice of his fantastic autobiography. One feels that some of his capers were so transparently false that he was mocking the staidness and pompousness which was now so characteristic of the British. But this impression is swiftly quashed an episode later when Prichard seems to be more pompous, more hypocritical, more zealous than even his contemporaries. His practice thrived because the gullible are everywhere; but his colleagues couldn't tolerate him. Nobody could empty a bar quicker than Pritchard; and Pritchard was the only one not to notice it. Although he had the qualifications for entry he couldn't get into the Faculty of Physicians and Surgeons because no Fellow would sponsor him; but he had success, short success, in getting into the Glasgow Athenaeum and the Society of Arts, whose members were soon rueing the day.

Pritchard's overbearing vanity soon had him lecturing on his adventures in far-flung exotic places, with the Royal Navy. He had little or no battle experience because naval warfare was in the doldrums following Nelson's defeat of Napoleon, but Pritchard found other attractions. There were graphic stories of his fights with savages and wild animals, of the like which wouldn't be seen again until the fictional adventures of Tarzan were published.

The accounts were so contradictory and so improbable that they couldn't even be called lies. So preposterous did Pritchard's behaviour become that he was often seen parading about with a walking stick on which had been engraved *To my good friend Dr. Pritchard from his friend General Garibaldi*. Garibaldi, the liberator of Italy, was an international hero at the time and Pritchard was claiming an intimacy with him. Apart from the fact that he knew hardly anything about the general and couldn't describe him, everybody had seen Pritchard with the stick before it was engraved.

He became a Knight Templar in the Glasgow Priory and joined the Grand Lodge of the Freemasons in Edinburgh where he began to flaunt himself in the costumes and medals of the office. It was soon discovered that his motives were self-interest and self-advertisement, which were directly opposite to the principles of Freemasonry.

He tried for a high position, the Andersonian Chair of Surgery at Edinburgh University, and backed up his application form with signed testimonials from the leading dozen surgeons in Britain, none of whom had ever heard of Pritchard. He never got the job, and nobody wasted time prosecuting him.

It is possible to detect a gradual deterioration in Pritchard, with his actions becoming more bizarre and irresponsible and since the same pattern is discernible in Dr. Cream, and several other doctors in this book, one wonders how far their weak personalities might have been further thrown off balance by drug addiction.

The first mysterious death involving Dr. Pritchard occurred in May 1863. Even though there were five lusty children romping around the house, as well as Mrs. Pritchard and the servants, the doctor didn't hesitate at taking a nip at one of the younger Nippies, and a girl was found dead in an upstairs bedroom after a fire gutted several rooms. Dr. Pritchard told the police that he had been out most of the evening and only discovered the fire moments after his return. There had only been time, he said, to raise his young sons, sleeping on the first floor and carry them to safety before the fire got out of hand. His wife and eldest children were away he said, so apart from a young maid there was nobody else in the home. They all went looking for the girl. She was found, partly burnt, on her bed in the room where the fire had started. What puzzled the police was the fact that she had made no attempt to escape. She lay in the centre of the bed as if peacefully sleeping. It was assumed that she had been asphyxiated before she could escape, as police doubted she would look so comfortable in the process of a painful death. Her body and facial muscles were relaxed and revealed no indication of any fight to save herself. Since the fire started in a corner, more-over, she should have had time to reach the door. The only explanation could be that she had been dead or unconscious when the fire started. Pritchard had the habit, when returning to the house, of checking to see if any patients had left him messages. On just one night, the night of the fire, he hadn't gone up to check – the very night when the girl would be fighting for her life.

The police found it downright suspicious and so did the in-surance company when Pritchard claimed for jewellery and property of which they could find not the merest trace in the gutted rooms.

Nothing was done. The girl was from the poor and inarticulate class and there was nobody to challenge the facts for her. The girl isn't even named in the subsequent evidence which was gathered for Pritchard's trial. Nobody could see any reason, at the time, why Pritchard, a respectable gentleman if somewhat eccentric, should destroy a girl. And assuming that he had been carrying out an abortion, and it had misfired, would the girl's features have shown such tranquil calmness? We mustn't forget the fact that she died at an opportune moment when Mrs. Pritchard and the eldest of her children were away. Since we have no evidence she was in the house, we must assume it was the cook's night off and she was the only other servant in the house.

Since Pritchard soon had an affair going with the girl who replaced the dead servant, we might as well assume, since it can't do him any harm, that he had an affair with the dead one. By Whit Sunday 1864, Dr. Pritchard had moved house to Sauchiehal Street, also in Glasgow, and was having an affair with the maid, Mary McLeod. Even Pritchard couldn't expect to get away with this sort of thing forever, especially as he was now reckless in his irresponsibility. Apparently he made love to Mary at a moment when he shouldn't have and Mrs. Pritchard, bouncing into the room, caught him in a "position vile and un-Victorian."

We have to leave it to our imaginations to speculate how Pritchard got out of that one. McLeod, however, not only found herself remaining with the family, but about to begin one, and Pritchard, obliging, had carried out an illegal operation for her. Perhaps she told him "do that three times and you must make me thine", for Pritchard told her about this time, she testified, "That if Mrs. Pritchard died before he and I did, he would marry me."

It was in the October of this very year that Mary Jane's health began to cause concern. And it had nothing to do with the time that she discovered Mary McLeod on her knees and her husband helping her to say her prayers. Mrs. Pritchard not only looked bad she felt bad. The pain she was suffering was abominable and left her terribly depressed. She suffered a loss of appetite, and a constant tendency to vomit caused her so much embarrassment that she retired to her bedroom.

Her mysterious illness remained until the end of November, and she had recovered sufficiently by the first weeks of December to go with her eldest daughter to stay (for a time) with her parents in Edinburgh. Pritchard had let her live long enough to enjoy Christmas. She returned to Glasgow for the holiday season but shortly after the New Year was struck down again. The symptoms and the sickness had returned with such a violence that she was heard to remark, more than once, "It's strange I'm all right in Edinburgh, and I'm ill in Glasgow."

His wife's illness gave Pritchard his shiniest hypocritical hour. All the neighbours murmured his praises as he, tirelessly, soft-footed it from the kitchen to the sick-room with broth and other light foods for "my beloved Mary Jane." The wife who was slowly wasting away, and in excruciating pain, was deluged in honeyed words each of which carried a gold-coloured exclamation mark. With the words came kisses, carefully planted on the feverish brow so as not to bruise.

Nobody had more conceit about his abilities and his appearance than Pritchard but where his wife's health was concerned, he maintained, he couldn't assume he knew it all, and he sought a second opinion on her illness. Whether this was a ruse, not uncommon with a poisoning doctor who can later claim, after the funeral, that he consulted his peers, or whether it was at the suggestion of his wife, we don't know. We do know he wrote to Dr. James Moffat Cowan, who lived in Edinburgh, and who was a distant relative of his wife. Dr. Cowan made the journey to Glasgow and found the patient in a better condition than Pritchard's high-flown prose had led him to suspect. Even this could be a ruse, a show of over-anxiousness because the patient was the woman for whom he cared. Pritchard said he thought his "darling Mary Jane" had an irritation of the stomach. Dr. Cowan seemed to concur and prescribed mustard poultices and glasses of champagne. Cowan left and Pritchard increased the antimony doses. Mrs Pritchard's condition deteriorated.

Pritchard now sought a third opinion, calling in a Dr. Gairdner. He said he thought that his wife was suffering from catalepsy, a trance inducing disease. Dr. Gairdner found Mrs. Pritchard highly excited and came to the conclusion she was intoxicated. Dr. Pritchard agreed and blamed Dr. Cowan for recommending champagne. Dr. Gairdner suggested a simple diet and no medicines. After a second visit, Pritchard didn't call him in again. If Mrs. Pritchard had asked him to consult other doctors, which is a possibility, it looks as if Pritchard was putting her off by telling her that Cowan and Gairdner were quacks and charlatans.

But the lack of faith was mutual. It seems that neither doctor had been impressed by Pritchard's show of husbandly affection or his medical knowledge. Both took action. But, to be fair to them, neither could have thought Pritchard worse than incompetent. They didn't suspect the truth, only doubted his ability. Back in Edinburgh, Dr. Cowan had called on Mrs. Taylor, Mary Jane's mother. He suggested she hurry to Glasgow and take care of her daughter. This strong and healthy old lady – despite her seventy years – caught the next train to Glasgow. She little knew that her own death was but two weeks away.

Meanwhile Dr. Gairdner was writing to Mary Jane's brother, Dr. Michael Taylor, who had a practice at Penrith. He roundly suggested that Mary Jane be taken to Penrith and put under her brother's care. One can imagine, especially by this second action, what effect Pritchard's behaviour and conversation must have had on these two members of his own profession. Dr. Taylor seemed sufficiently alarmed to write suggesting that Mary Jane be sent to him. Shrewdly, Dr. Pritchard didn't refuse the suggestion. He delayed, saying that Mary Jane wasn't sufficiently well yet to travel.

Mrs. Taylor was a character and Pritchard expressed a great affection for her. It was she who had helped buy his practices and his homes. It might be that she regarded him as a bit of a problem, but she was fond of him. Pritchard, however, saw her arrival as a threat and he turned to face the new danger. He marked time on the destruction of his wife, while he demolished the mother first. In the meantime, he kept up his great play of affection, spreading kisses and soft words in all directions. He was buying large supplies of antimony and aconite. "I never furnished so much poison to one medical man," a chemist was to observe. In a few weeks Pritchard had purchased more antimony than all other Glasgow doctors together did in a year. To show what Pritchard thought of Mrs. Taylor, we have a letter that he had recently written to his eldest daughter, who was staying with his mother-in-law in Edinburgh.

"Kiss dear grandmother for me," he wrote. "Love her and help her all you can, and when the rolling years pass away you will remember my advice and be happier far by doing so than I can positively make you understand now. Pray to our Heavenly Father quietly and alone to spare her to us, to protect you from all harm, and to make you a good girl and, in due time, a Christian woman, and a blessing to us all. Never forget kind friends, those who have an interest in your well-being."

With the ink hardly dry on these sickly words, Pritchard turned from the slow and painful murdering of his wife to the killing of her mother.

The eldest daughter, incidentally, seemed to spend a lot of time with her grandparents. She was very fond of her father and would eventually visit him daily in jail. Just prior to his execution she would write a pathetic letter to the prison officials asking them to be kind to poor papa. One wonders if Mrs. Pritchard left her in Edinburgh because of her illness. Or, more probably, because she was frightened that the girl might catch *poor papa* plastered against Mary McLeod delivering the kiss of life.

Grandmother Taylor arrived in Glasgow on the Friday, by the Monday she had been stricken down. Between fits of vomiting, she observed, "It looks as if I've got Mary Jane's malady."

Dr. Pritchard declared that he had discovered the reason for her illness. It seems Granny took great dollops of a tonic called *Battley's Sedative Solution*. Bottles of this type of pick-me-up sold in millions to temperate Victorians who fooled themselves into believing that they were indeed taking medicine and not alcohol or drugs. Granny stood by *Battley's* which was laced with opium, and she was never without it. Soon Pritchard was whispering to visitors behind his hand and heavily winking: "The old lady likes her drop, you know."

What had actually felled Mrs. Taylor was tapioca. Mrs. Pritchard had asked for some, and it had been cooked and taken to the dining room. It hadn't been intended for her mother who had sampled some after Pritchard had tampered with it.

But since Granny was up and briskly about in a day or so it seems likely that, at this time, Pritchard didn't intend her any harm. The presumption is that she began to suspect something of the truth over the next few days, and Pritchard decided that she had to go. On February 24, a former cook to the household called to take the children for a walk and Granny expressed her anxiety to this woman about her daughter's health. She said she was completely baffled by the illness and writing letters in all directions – presumably to doctors she knew – to try and diagnose the cause.

On this day, Granny sent Mary McLeod to get her some sausages for dinner and the skinned mysteries brought her crashing down after she had eaten them. She had taken to spending all day with her daughter and sleeping in her room at night. She had just got back there after eating the sausages when she became violently sick. Also staying in the house were two male students and Pritchard promptly sent one of these for a Dr. Paterson, who lived nearby, because he said he was mystified by his mother-in-law's illness and wanted a second opinion.

Dr. Paterson, who was to emerge badly from the affair at the subsequent trial, claimed he suspected the truth as soon as he entered the sick-room. Granny had been lifted from the floor where she had collapsed on to the bed beside her daughter. Dr. Paterson thought she had been dosed with a powerful narcotic and was dying.

Pritchard, it seems, had waylaid him in the hall and told him that she liked a drop of the hard stuff, but Paterson knew she had taken more than a dram of drink. He also saw Mrs. Pritchard for the first time since her illness and he was shocked by the sight of her. She was sitting up beyond her mother in a state of pitiful agitation and distress, and looking so pale and wasted that she seemed almost dead. Dr. Paterson thought, he later said, that she was under the influence of antimony, a strong depressant.

Paterson found Mrs. Taylor unconscious and breathing heavily. Mrs. Pritchard, with weak voice and weak arms, was trying pitifully to arouse her mother. Dr. Pritchard hopped about the room calling to God to help. When his mother-in-law, for a moment, regained consciousness, Pritchard slapped her shoulder and shouted at her, "You are getting better, darling!"

Dr. Paterson answered for her. "Never in this world," he said grimly.

Pritchard now confessed to Paterson that Granny was addicted to *Battley's*, which, as he knew, contained opium. He said she had just recently purchased a half-pound bottle – she had sent Mary McLeod for it – and Pritchard now told Dr. Paterson, "It's probable she's taken a good swig of it."

Dr. Paterson left, convinced that Mrs. Taylor would shortly die. He also left with the conviction that Mrs. Pritchard was being poisoned – but he did nothing about it. His excuse at the trial, when he was savaged by lawyers, was that he hadn't been asked for an opinion on Mrs. Pritchard, who was the patient of her husband, and it therefore it wasn't his business. Later that night, Dr. Paterson was summoned to see Mrs. Taylor again, but, considering the case hopeless, he decided not to go. Mrs. Taylor died in a coma at one o'clock in the morning, and Pritchard hopped along to his study to record the facts while they were still fresh in his diary. He said:

> "About 1 a.m. this morning passing away calmly – peacefully – and the features retaining a life-like character – so finely drawn was the transition that it would be impossible to determine with decision the moment when life may be said to be departed."

If Pritchard, perhaps to sake his conscience, wasn't actually saying Mrs. Taylor looked better dead than alive, he was saying

that there was no difference in her and therefore nothing untoward had happened. He was back in the death room when the
two servants were laying Mrs. Taylor out and he sprung at the
bottle of *Battley's* which had been in the pocket of her smock.
He waved it angrily as if it was the culprit, then delivered some
of his exclamation-marked sentences. "Good Heavens!" he
screamed. "Has she swallowed all this since Tuesday!"

He swore the servants to secrecy on the amount she had taken,
implanting in their simple minds, for the sake of any future
inquiry, the idea that the tonic had killed the old lady. He told
them they must think of her good reputation and his, for his
practice would suffer if it was discovered that he had permitted
his mother-in-law to drink such copious amounts of such a lethal
brew. "We have a sad house today," he was soon observing to
visitors.

A few days later Dr. Paterson met Pritchard in the street.
Pritchard asked him to look in on his wife on the following day
because he was going to Edinburgh for his mother-in-law's
funeral. Dr. Paterson would testify that he called on Mrs.
Pritchard and that his first impression – that she was being
poisoned by antimony – was confirmed. Yet he gave no warning
to the poor woman, said nothing to Pritchard about his suspicions, nor did he discuss the matter with anybody else.

In Edinburgh, Mr. Taylor ran into problems in burying his
wife. Pritchard told him it would be unethical for him to sign
the death certificate because she had been Dr. Paterson's patient.
The widower caught the train to Glasgow, called on Dr.
Paterson, and discovered Paterson wouldn't sign it. Paterson's
behaviour is odd. The best you can say for him is that he was a
coward and didn't wish to get himself involved. He wouldn't be
specific to the widower about his refusal to sign the certificate,
but would only say it was contrary to medical etiquette.

Pritchard had already alerted the authorities to the fact that
Mrs. Taylor was Paterson's patient, for Paterson received a
document to fill in from the authorities. He wrote back to the
registrar saying he refused to sign the document because Mrs.
Taylor's death was *sudden, unexpected, and mysterious.* Before the
registrar could give some thought to this, however, a death
certificate arrived. Mr. Taylor had gone back to Edinburgh, seen
Pritchard, and Pritchard had signed it. The document showed
his usual incompetence for he put "primary cause of death,
paralysis for a duration of twelve hours; secondary cause,
apoplexy for a duration of one hour." No skilled doctor would
put the causes in this order but would reverse them because
apoplexy precedes paralysis.

With his mother-in-law out of the way, Pritchard now resumed destroying his wife. She was eating very little food now, but what she was eating, Pritchard was bringing her. Visitors reported her as being a shadow of her former self. She was fading away. They found her in pain, weak, thin and depressed.

"It's strange," she said wistfully to some of these people, "that I'm always well in Edinburgh and ill in Glasgow."

Dr. Pritchard might be busy in the surgery and the sick-room; he might also be busy with Mary McLeod and one or two of his love-lorn patients, but he managed to hammer out some correspondence. His daughter and father-in-law were deluged with letters describing the frantic fight he was putting up so that "our Mary Jane" and "our darling mother" would soon be well and back with them all again. When pretentious phrases deserted him, which was rare, he fell back on to Holy Writ. Since Dr. Michael Taylor might pose some threat from Penrith, letters flowed to him, minutely detailing Mary Jane's symptoms and the treatment he was giving her.

If brother Michael then thought that there was nothing unduly wrong with Mary Jane and that much of her illness was only in Dr. Pritchard's mind because of his deep affection for his wife, who could blame him for not hurrying to Glasgow?

On March 17, the cook, Mary Paterson, was in the kitchen when she heard the bell sound in the sick-room. It was midday. The bell sounded a second time and then a third time, violently. Mary Paterson hurried up to the ground floor, wondering where Mary McLeod was, since it was her duty to answer the summons. She saw the door to the consulting room slightly open, and she pushed it. It wouldn't budge. Somebody was obviously behind it, holding it there.

Good servants keep their thoughts to themselves, and if Mary Paterson theorised as to what was going on behind the door, she never mentioned it. She had only gone a few paces when the consulting room door opened. Dr. Pritchard appeared: "How is Mrs. Pritchard!" he barked. Mary Paterson said she was answering the bell to find out. The doctor followed her upstairs and from behind the doctor suddenly appeared Mary McLeod. The delay had probably been occasioned by the fact that the couple had had to adjust their dress.

Mary Paterson left the sick-room for a moment. When she returned the doctor was giving his wife a drink from a porter-sized glass. Later in the afternoon, Mary was to testify, Mrs. Pritchard became light-headed. She talked to her mother as if she was alive and in the room. She also suffered from severe cramp.

Her condition worsened, and Pritchard sent for his old ally, Dr. Paterson. Dr. Paterson, who had missed the chance to tell Mr. Taylor about his suspicions on his wife's death and the fact that his daughter was probably being poisoned by antimony; who had also missed the opportunity to talk to the registrar and the police, was now astonished by the deterioration he now saw in Mrs. Pritchard. He hadn't seen her for fifteen days.

Mrs. Pritchard told him she hadn't slept for four or five days, but Pritchard disputed this. He told Paterson to take little heed of what his wife said because she was delerious. Now was the moment to face Pritchard and tell him what he suspected, but Paterson did not do so. All that he suggested was a sleeping draught. Pritchard said there was none in the house so Paterson dictated a prescription to Pritchard, which the latter signed. Dr. Paterson then left – for the last time.

Pritchard and Mary McLeod stayed in the sickroom. Pritchard curled up on the bed beside his wife, holding her hand while the maid rested on the sofa. She had been instructed by Pritchard to fetch a poultice at one o'clock, and she left to do this. She woke the cook, Mary Paterson, and returning to treat Mrs. Pritchard with the poultice, and found her dead. Dr. Pritchard refused to believe it. He demanded hot water to restore her animation. Mary Paterson said, "Water would be no use to a dead body, sir." Pritchard looked startled on these words. He was warming up for his big scene. "Is she dead, Paterson?"

When the woman confirmed it, Pritchard smote his chest and held his hand above his brow. He cried out, "Come back! Come back, my dear Mary Jane. I beg you, don't leave your dear Edward!" He also added, mysteriously: "What a brute! What a heathen!" They weren't sure who he was talking about but then it seemed that he was referring to himself, for he asked Mary Paterson to fetch a rifle which was in the house and shoot him. The servants assumed he was blaming himself for not curing his wife.

Pritchard then shot off to write letters and bring his diary up to date with the latest death. He wrote in the diary:

> "Died here at 1 a.m. Mary Jane, my own beloved wife, aged 38 – no torment surrounded her bedside – but, like a calm, peaceful lamb of God – passed Minnie away. May God and Jesus, Holy Ghost, one in three – welcome Minnie. Prayer on prayer till mine be o'er; ever-lasting love. Save us, Lord, for Thy dear Son."

There would be more opportunities for melodramatics before Mary Jane was buried; at the station when the coffin was put on the train for Edinburgh; at his father-in-law's house where he would rip off the coffin lid for one more kiss from those cold lips; at the grave-side where he would have to be held so as to save himself from injury as he tried to crash into the grave. But in the meantime, with his wife freshly dead, Pritchard busied himself with his letters. He hurried out in the early hours to post these. He came back excited from this mission and called Mary Paterson up from the kitchen. The ghost of his wife had walked up the street with him, he declared, and begged him before she left, to take care of their daughters. She hadn't mentioned their sons, however, and Pritchard wondered about this. But, he told the cook, she had kissed him on the cheek before disappearing.

One of the important letters was to his bank concerning a complaint of theirs about his overdraft, which was £131. Although he used the deaths as an excuse for not attending to it, it is inconceivable that the motives for both murders was merely to get a delay in settling this matter. He wrote to the bank:

> "I am fully aware of the overdraft, and nothing short of the heavy affliction I have been visited with since the year commencing in the loss of my mother, and this day my wife, after long and severe illness, would have made me break my promise. If you will kindly tell Mr. Readman, to whom I am well known, that immediately I can attend to business I will see him on the matter. Please ask him if he can wait till after my dear wife's funeral on Thursday."

No clear motive is discernible in Pritchard's crimes and baffled, his contemporaries, hesitantly, point to this overdraft and the fact that Pritchard stood to collect a two-thirds return on an interest from an investment on his wife's death. But the capital was only £2,500 to begin with, and Pritchard couldn't hope to collect more than £50, if that, in a year. Since this would, in any case, have gone to Mrs. Pritchard before her death, he would already be receiving the benefit from it.

We have no reason to disbelieve Mary McLeod that Pritchard, in a moment of passion, promised her marriage should his wife die; but it is harder to believe that the doctor, a notorious dandy and snob, would take an unlettered serving girl about with him as his wife. Since Mrs. Pritchard hadn't ordered Mary from the house when she caught them, in the middle of their love-making, and since he was still enjoying the girl's favours, she would hardly seem to qualify as a motive for murder. Dr. Cross, as we see elsewhere, murdered his wife because she sacked their governess after catching the two of them making love. On the other hand, Mrs. Pritchard seems to have tolerated the affair.

We can't know all the facts. It could be possible that Pritchard had high hopes elsewhere. He was only forty, and women found him both handsome and charming, especially women of the more fluttery and butterfly sort. He had a great many women patients, among them well-off widows and daughters from wealthy homes. It is more than probable that one of these had shown a liking for him, a liking which could develop into something much stronger if he weren't encumbered with a wife. Since divorce was hard to come by, expensive, and beyond the attainment of a doctor, who needed respectability, it could be that Pritchard, not the first man to decide so, came to the conclusion that poison was the only way out.

It would have pleased Pritchard's pronounced vanity to have an attractive wife instead of the careworn one that Mary Jane had become, and if she brought a dowry with her he would no longer need to worry about mundane things like overdrafts and even the undoubted hard work which was involved in running a medical practice. His notorious incompetence points to a disenchantment with his work. So he set out to murder his wife, but first, because she got in the way, he had to remove Mrs. Taylor. Smooth Pritchard might have been, but nor did they come any rougher than he.

Pritchard was arrested as he stepped from the train at Glasgow after returning from his wife's funeral in Edinburgh, where he had shed so many tears it looked like rain. It had been an anonymous letter received by the authorities, which had started the hunt. Everybody later said that Dr. Paterson's conscience had been worrying him so much that he had sent it, but this he denied.

While Pritchard, then, was scattering tears like confetti in Edinburgh, the police were doing overtime in Glasgow. So confident were they, it seemed, that they arrested Pritchard before his house had been searched or before any post mortem could be carried out on Mrs. Taylor and his wife. Perhaps they had discovered the great amounts of antimony that he had brought, and had decided that, for the moment, this was evidence enough.

Pritchard made a good impression on nearly everybody he spoke to after his arrest, and he also impressed the court. His smile, while sad because of his recent bereavement, was sufficient to indicate that he had nothing to hide or fear. His beard was neatly trimmed and pomaded. He was as usual, well-dressed and was calm, thoughtful, and, for once, modest. He won immediate public support for there was, really, no true evidence to suggest murder. Confident of his innocence, his own family stood by him. They thought it all a misunderstanding and that he would soon be released. Surprisingly, Pritchard thought this too. He went on thinking it even after a post mortem on his wife was ordered. The first tests were negative and chemists were called in to carry out a further post mortem.

Pritchard was still serenely confident. Then came the shattering news on March 28. Mary Jane's body was deluged with antimony. The chemists found so much poison in her organs that the wonder was that she had held on to life for so long. Pritchard still pleaded innocence and bafflement. "Who could have done such a dastardly thing!" he demanded to know. The ham actor in him came to the fore and the authorities were sufficiently impressed to believe him when he produced his theory; if anybody killed poor Mary Jane, Pritchard was soon declaring, it had to be the maid Mary McLeod. To the men of the world around him he blushingly, and ashamedly, admitted all.

In a moment of weakness he had yielded to the temptations of the flesh, (notably Mary McLeod's flesh), which she had brazenly tempted him with. Well, one thing had led to another. After all, with his mother-in-law, and then his wife ill, he had been forced to turn to somebody for comfort and succour. Yes, Dr. Pritchard was certain of it. The illiterate maid had obtained the poison and dosed his wife in the crazy belief that, with his wife dead, the doctor would marry her.

The authorities then interrogated Mary McLeod. She confessed what little she knew – and it was very little. The doctor had seduced her; had aborted her once; and had promised her marriage should his wife die. Nothing more. It was obvious that the girl hadn't poisoned Mary Jane, or been involved in the plot but, because it was the only out they had, the defence kept up this line of argument during the trial. The judge contemptuously dismissed the suggestion – as did the jury.

With nobody else to turn to Pritchard turned to God, or at least seemed too. No official was so lowly in office that he didn't attempt to impress him with his shining goodness. Footsteps outside the door of his cell would send Pritchard crashing to his knees, all the while sending up a feverish prayer.

Astonishingly enough the police and prison officers, used to the wiles of criminals, were impressed by Pritchard. They liked him, and not only because he was ever-ready to ask them, if they had a spare moment, to join him on his knees in instant prayer.

Most people, initially, were impressed by Pritchard, of course, and he wasn't around the prison long enough before they hanged him, for his insincerity to become sickingly apparent. He wept so copiously in court when his wife or his mother-in-law were mentioned that the cleaners found the floor ready scrubbed. And yet he showed an unconcern as he smiled at the judges and prosecution lawyers as if, by winning them over, he thought he might get a release, with just a warning not to do such things again.

The defence had an uphill task, but they battled on manfully. Pritchard was a gentleman; there had been two admirals in his family, and gentlemen just didn't do the things Pritchard had been charged with. This was the kernel of the defence's attack. But Mary McLeod, with her eyes on a distinguished and handsome husband, might well murder, they suggested. To get from gutter to palace was her motive. Gentlemen didn't do such things, but Pritchard undoubtedly had, which confirmed what a lot of people had felt for a long time: that he was no gentleman.

The jury eventually came to the same conclusion. It was noticed that the defence produced no character witnesses on Pritchard's behalf. Colleagues who wouldn't vote him into medical clubs were hardly likely to give him a character reference while he was being tried for murder.

There was no defence, but only Pritchard seemed surprised when he was found guilty and sentenced to death. His capacity for self-delusion suggested either perpetual intoxication or insanity. Under pressure from a bevy of clergymen, it took him three attempts before he could commit to paper the fact that he had destroyed his mother-in-law, whom he seemed to have looked on with as much affection as if she had been his own mother. Since he couldn't now give out photo portraits of himself, Pritchard scribbled out texts from Scriptures and issued these instead.

Almost royal in his arrogance, he issued a sort of proclamation in which he mentioned people he wished to thank for their kindnesses or services. The name of his counsel, who hadn't saved him, was omitted from the list. Pritchard had no time for failures. He blocked the publication of his confession until after his execution, determined people should think good of him until the end.

He was calm and composed at his execution, the last publicly held one in Glasgow, if not in Scotland, and a hundred thousand people turned up to see him off. Pritchard was sure he was heading for Heaven, for a meeting with his dear Mary Jane and mother-in-law. "We shall meet again in Heaven," he told the clergyman who accompanied him to the scaffold. That good man, although reluctant to be a carrier of bad tidings at such a moment, nevertheless, felt compelled to be accurate. He corrected, "No, sir, but at the Judgement Seat."

DR. HERMANN WEBSTER MUDGETT

Scratch an American for his list of the *all time greats* in American crime and he will invariably give you a list of gun-toters like Billy the Kid, Jesse James, John Dillinger and Al Capone. But probably only one in a hundred will mention Dr. Hermann Webster Mudgett, or H. H. Holmes, as he became known. He was a rat-like little man, with weak eyes and buck-teeth, a way with women, a walrus moustache, and an undertaker's habit of always dressing in black. Although he is hardly known by the man in the street today, no American murdered with greater panaché and confidence, or got more profit out of his victims. He even reduced them down to the bone and sold their skeletons to medical schools. His motives were sadistic and profit-seeking and he also displayed a tidiness of mind which is almost domestic, in that he wanted to get rid of one woman before he replaced her with the next.

Holmes built a home in Chicago in the style of a medieval castle but he ensured that it was equipped with modern rubbish disposal gadgets, in this instance a chute which could swiftly transport a corpse from the bedrooms above to the basement-dungeon below. The English must have looked across the Atlantic with envy when the facts concerning the diminutive doctor first reached the courts, for such furtive behaviour in the commission of crime was more of their style of work. Mayhem in murky, moated houses was European; traditionally American crime was open and accompanied by the lusty roar of a forty five. The English Victorians, testily and enviously, would have maintained that the Americans had no right to a mass murderer like Holmes. Their fears were justified by the obscurity Holmes dropped into once he had dropped through the hangman's trap floor. In England Holmes would have been taken to the national heart and put on an immortal pedestal beside Jack the Ripper. Many a melodrama would have been staged, and a pennydreadful printed about his exploits. Many a reverend gentleman would have galvanised his congregation by ascribing a like fate to any teenager before him, who wandered from the staid straight and sterile narrow.

Mudgett, or Holmes as he preferred to call himself, was born at Gilmanton, New Hampshire, in May 1860, the son of the local postmaster. He became a schoolmaster after his graduation and then studied medicine at Ann Arbor, obtaining a degree at the age of 24. He had married before this to Clara Lovering of Alton, and they had had a son. He deserted both in New York, where, for a time, he practised medicine. He next went to Chicago, he changed his name to Holmes, and bigamously married a girl named Myrta Belknapp.

Apparently before his mid-twenties Mudgett had a reputation of the kind that people furtively whispered about. Nothing you could actually come straight out with and prove. Reporters and detectives would catch up with the whispers at a much later date, after the damage was all done. There had been a student who had lost money and there had been another who mysteriously died. Then there was the cadaver that disappeared from a medical school but somehow had life insurance paid out on it under another name. But these whispers had been hard to substantiate so long after the fact and, in any case, the 'tecs had all they wanted for Homes's trial after they took his Chicago castle apart. In the squat, ugly, three-storey building they found a dungeon of sorts, a huge vat beneath the chute for reducing flesh and fat. There were cell-like rooms padded to deaden screams, and which were usually windowless. These were peculiarly furnished only with asbestos or steel-sheeting. Doors had secret peepholes just like conventional prison cells. The investigators therefore had all they wanted in the Chicago castle without having to dig back into the monster's greening years, and much we would like to know about this lady-killer went missing.

His bigamous marriage to Miss Belknapp didn't last long mainly because of the outrageous manner in which he tried to swindle the wealthy uncle of his defacto bride. This led to a family quarrel and a parting of the way. The "Black Baron" next worked for a widow named Mrs. Holden. Ostensibly it seemed he was hired to manage her drug store at Englewood, Chicago, but Holmes had soon moved into the domestic side of the property. Then, strangely and without announcement, Mrs. Holden vanished and Holmes seemed to have become owner of the thriving business. When friends asked for her whereabouts, he promptly said, "California – somewhere there." Although she never wrote, the friends never carried the matter further, perhaps because Holmes was such a mild and inoffensive little man, and nobody could imagine that he had done her in.

Holmes began to seduce girls who worked in the store. Old hands had dozens of stories of coming into the store unexpectedly and catching the boss at it. But he wasn't neglecting business apparently, accumulating and investing money. It was now he built his castle. It was on a piece of land facing the drug store and the ugly three-storey building looked as weird from the outside as it would from the interior. "Funny looking house," said a customer to Holmes once.

"It's not a house," Holmes corrected primly, "it's a castle."

In 1890 a jeweller named Conner settled in Englewood with his pretty wife Julia and Conner's equally attractive sister, Gertie. When Conner's wanted a corner of the store to set up a watch repair business, Holmes obliged and for rent he seems to have taken both Julia and Gertie as his mistresses. Having lost both a wife and a sister in the move, Conner left in disgust and later divorced Julia.

Gossip has it that Julia was a spoilt and demanding woman, and it appears she was soon complaining to the doctor, (who if he looked dominatable certainly wasn't), about his goings-on with sister-in-law Gertie and a new arrival, a slim teenager named Emily Van Tassell. One can only visualise the rumpus but we do know that Julia, this time, had her way, because neither Gertie nor Miss Van Tassell were seen again.

The castle seemed to be cleared for action now, the spring doors oiled, the bags of quicklime stored, the dissecting instruments at hand. Holmes ran his estate office from a room on the third floor. Outside his room sat a comely secretary. Holmes's secretaries not only had to do overtime after office hours, but they had the unnerving habit of vanishing suddenly. Next to the doctor's office was a bathroom, which had no window. Instead, there was a panel in the wall, which opened on to one of the two chutes. A body could therefore take a quick bath then a joy-ride to the cellar.

One secretary we do know a little about, was a statuesque blonde named Emmeline Cigrand. She was remembered as being sophisticated and confident, and soon told everybody she preferred to be called Amelia, not Emmeline. Julia took an instant dislike to Amelia, no doubt because she felt threatened It was an accurate prediction. Julia told Holmes that Amelia would have to go, Holmes apparently decided not yet, and Julia and her daughter disappeared instead. Amelia soon went too. We do know when and where because a prosecution witness was to say that he saw her laid out on a slab in the castle's basement, for processing down to bone.

This witness, aptly named Charles Chopman, had answered an advertisement in a local newspaper, which read: *Wanted. Skeleton articulator. Apply H. H. Holmes. 701 Sixty-third Street. After noon*. Chopman called and found a mild-mannered little runt of a man with weak eyes and a soft voice, who didn't seem the type who would say boo to a crippled goose, and certainly didn't strike him as a lady-killer in any sense of the phrase. Holmes treated Chopman with grave suspicion, and checked out every one of his references, before allowing him to get to work on the delectable corpse which waited in the dungeon. It was an old con-man's trick that not only put Chopman on his guard, but gave Holmes an undeserved halo of respectability.

Chopman's description of his first visit to the dungeon is macabrely comic. He was talking with the doctor in the book-lined lounge when the doctor said, "We'll go to work now." He walked to the wall, sprung a hidden button and the wall swung away on a silent fulcrum. Chopman said the cellar was dark and windowless. He saw the naked body of a beautiful girl laid out on a slab. She was blonde. He later identified her by photographs as Emmeline Cigrand because of a cleft in her chin. Holmes explained, "She died of heart failure. Pity. Such a beauty."

Chopman made some remark about the secrecy of it all, which brought the sarcastic response from Holmes, "This is the sort of work you can't do in a store window overlooking the street."

Chopman was still hesitant, apparently, and Holmes assured him that he needn't be frightened.

Holmes had already told Chopman that he supplied skeletons to medical schools, and this particular skeleton had been ordered by the Hahnemann Medical School. Like a commercial hunter, Holmes wasted nothing. The girl's jewellery and clothes were sold, and later, her bones. Had the pet food industry been commercially developed at the time, no doubt Holmes would have found a ready market for the flesh. The atmosphere seems to have given Chopman the creeps, and this before Hollywood horror movies could have given a boost to his imagination. The medieval trappings and the diminutive doctor in black somewhat unnerved Chopman, according to his later evidence. He knew where the lovely blonde was going, to the medical school, but he was troubled about from whence she came.

Holmes told him, "Don't worry. Everything's in order. Hahnemann wants the job done, so let's agree your fee."

Chopman asked for $36, and Holmes agreed without argument.

Given the impression that the body had come from the medical school, Chopman began chopping with Holmes watching him – watching with an absorbed interest and a quirky little smile on his lips. Chopman testified that Holmes became excited after a time, and rushed from the cellar, only to return with his own bag of instruments. Enthusiastically, he said, "Look, let me help." He had then thrown himself into the work with the nostalgic enthusiasm of an old medical student.

Chopman, a Chicago mechanic who later became an alcoholic, admitted to stripping three corpses down to bone. Two women – one man. He also indicated Holmes's style of torture for, with the exception of Amelia Cigrand, the corpses all had facial mutilations which seemed to be acid burns. One of the little doctor's tricks was to splash acid over the faces of his lovely victims. This after luring them into soundproofed rooms.

Several medical schools would eventually admit to buying skeletons from Holmes and a rough count put the tally at a dozen. But other victims seemed to have been rendered to nothing in the cellar's lime-pit before Holmes realised that there was profit to be made in bones. The question springs to mind as to why Holmes needed Chopman at all. He was creating a danger by bringing in a witness to do a job he had demonstrated he could do himself. Moreover Holmes, who has left obvious evidence of his meanness, was reducing his profits from the medical schools by paying Chopman part of the fees.

But Holmes would have no fears on the score that he was creating potentially dangerous witnesses. He fooled better men, and women, than Chopman. When Julia wrote to friends in Davenport, Iowa, that she was going to marry a doctor who would invest several thousand dollars on her behalf, the friends weren't troubled when they never heard from Julia again. Nor, does it appear that the ex-husband, Mr. Conner, was concerned unduly by the disappearance of his ex-wife and their young daughter.

It is almost certain that some of these people came looking for friends and relatives who were last known to be staying at Holmes Castle. Yet time after time, the soft and weak-looking little doctor with the suave grave-side manner dispelled any suspicions these seekers might have had. We can only imagine what stories he told a mother or a father, a sister or brother, about a missing girl. Did he look mournful and sprout a tear and say the girl had left him for another, sort of gone West to the wide open spaces? Even several men who Holmes employed around his castle, although somewhat suspicious by the goings-on they noticed, ignored the awful truth.

An Irishman, one Patrick Quinlan, wouldn't believe the evidence of his own eyes. Later he said, "I left because the job gave me nightmares. The doctor had women all over the house. He had them in every room. Then, suddenly, they would vanish."

The Irishman was followed by a black named Henry Owens.

"It was more like a Moslem's harem than a Norman keep," he told reporters. Owens had the distinction of nearly being strangled by the doctor. He said, "I opened a door and found the doc busy with a girl. They were making love. I hurriedly backed out and slammed the door. I made noises of apology. But suddenly the doc came rushing out in a rage, jumped me from the rear, and nearly throttled me. Then he recovered and said it wasn't my fault since I had every right to go in the room at that time of day, and laughed and walked away." Owens added, "But the doc was so unlike his usual gentle self that it really scared me."

He couldn't name the girl, but said she was one of the doctor's secretaries. The reason why he couldn't name her he said, was that the doctor changed his secretaries so quickly, "But like all of them," he added, "she was beautiful."

Holmes sold the Holden drugstore towards the end of 1892 and moved permanently into his medieval stronghold. In May 1893, the Chicago World Fair opened and until October, the windy city was thronged with visitors. Since hotel space was at a premium, Holmes turned a useful dollar by letting some of the rooms in his castle. Rumour later had it that some of his guests disappeared. Be that true or false, by now Holmes had a mistress who was openly declaring herself to be his wife. She was a blonde heiress from Fort Worth, Texas, named Minnie Williams. She was to disappear with $20,000 of her money. But before she went, her sister, Nannie, disappeared.

Holmes told Minnie, "Why don't you have Nannie pay us a visit?"

The coming but not the going of Nannie was noticed but since Minnie lasted another six months, the grotesque theory was later broached that Minnie had connived with the doctor at her own sister's murder.

Before Minnie went the way of all Holmes flesh however, there was a fire in the castle. There had been other mysterious fires pointing to arson, for insurance, in Holmes's past. It happened in November, a month after the Fair closed and the tourists no longer needed rooms.

Like everything about Holmes, the affair of the fire continues in character, and contains features which are unbelievable. The insurance men came to assess the damage done to several rooms and Minnie Williams, inadvertently or deliberately, let slip the fact that it was arson. If Holmes seems unreal as he comes down to us, like something invented in medieval Hungary by peasants to frighten their children to sleep, what about his victims, like Minnie, and what about the people who investigated him and presumably did nothing when they discovered a crime?

The insurance company didn't pay for the damage, but they didn't do anything else either.

The month of November was a busy one for our Black Baron. There was the fire and Minnie's indiscretions, which meant Minnie had to go. So Minnie went. It seems she was scheduled to leave at this time, in any case, for Holmes also got married in November, down towards the end of the month. It was an exception these days for Holmes to marry, but this he did to Georgina Yoke from Indiana, and it was said she won him because she refused him the fruit of love without a band of gold. No sweat perhaps for Holmes who had his own swift and brutally effective ways of divorcing. Shortly after this, he was arrested on some obscure fraud charge, and the new wife hastened to do her wifey duty and bail him out.

We know by the evidence what his help thought about his activities, though they did nothing more than worry about it; but what did his neighbours think with this steady traffic of delectable females to, but never from, the medieval castle down the street? One wonders their reaction in the first place, to the great ugly pile stuck right next door. Even without knowing about the chutes, peepholes and padded cells. No doubt males in the district were kind of envious of the doc's penchant for pulling dolls. But they must have comforted themselves with such lines as *He can't keep them for long, don't ya notice? Yeah, they're soon off looking for a real man.* And later, when the truth would out, as it sometimes does. *Little Doc Holmes with those weak eyes and pudgy hands, a killer? I don't believe it. Never in a million years.*

Holmes's very nondescript appearance was an ally. He looked the very epitome of spineless, overfed, under-exercised, dehydrated, gone-to-seed, never-had-it suburban man. If anybody could have made looking like an undersized slob pay, it was Holmes. Murderers just didn't look like him. Murderers were hulking brutes with banana-shaped fingers, muscles like coconuts and bad breath.

Had he continued in his traditional way, murdering his secretaries and cashing in on their skeletons, it seems Holmes, in the safety of his castle, could have gone on forever. But he was married now and that might well have been the reason for his change. Perhaps he was genuinely in love and had given up all other women with the arrival of Indiana's Miss Yoke. Whatever the reason the Black Baron sought his future victims and profit outside the safety of his castle. If his past had all the ingredients from which medieval fairy stories are made, the scheme he now mounted had all the improbabilities of a bad movie script. The ham actor, which Holmes undoubtedly was, conspired with the mad Machiavellian in his twisted mind to evolve a plot which would involve the destruction of a confederate, and which would scatter that unfortunate man's family, also murdered, across several states. The caper had its beginning in Philadelphia, and Holmes would have got away with the crime but for the suspicions of a Philadelphian police detective named Frank Geyer.

On a dull September morning detective Frank Geyer got a routine order to check a death at number 1316 Callowhill Street. He did not know that he was setting out on what was to prove his most baffling and greatest case and one which would lead to the exposure of a mass murderer. Earlier, a carpenter named Eugene Smith had found Mr. Perry, an inventor, dead on the floor of his laboratory. Geyer arrived at the shabby building and while looking for the right floor noticed a canvas sign saying *B. F. Perry, Patents Bought and Sold.*

Geyer found Smith waiting there with a man – who lay dead on the floor. A man who wore trousers of a peculiarly milk chocolate colour. There were burn marks on the wall and bits of glass scattered about. The man's face was badly burnt by acid, so much so that Eugene Smith said he could hardly recognise him as his friend. Smith thought that Perry had been smoking his pipe, and there was a corncob lying nearby, and that when it had gone out he had stupidly relit it and caused an explosion. There was even a dead match stick near the body.

It looked at first glance like a straight forward accident to Geyer, but he had pieces of glass and other equipment taken away for examination. An autopsy showed that Perry's lungs were seared. But the scientists could only confirm what Geyer already knew, that an explosion had taken place and Perry had inhaled acid which had killed him. Geyer had already decided that Smith had been wrong on one point. The tobacco in the pipe was unscorched so it looked as if the inventor hadn't foolishly caused the explosion by striking a match.

Geyer had an uneasy feeling about the death but as there was nothing he could put his finger on, he shelved it at the back of his mind to cogitate on when he had a spare moment. The dead man seemed to have had no friends and no money so the authorities paid for the funeral. It was on the very day of the funeral that the Fidelity Mutual Life Association of Philadelphia received a letter at their Walnut Street headquarters from Chicago. The letter, from a solicitor named Jeptha D. Howe, said:

> "B. F. PERRY is, in my opinion, actually Benjamin F. Pitezel of Chicago, who last September took out a policy in your company naming his wife, Carrie A. Pitezel, also of this

city as beneficiary. Mr. Pitezel has for some time been in financial difficulties, and it was for that reason that he went to another city and took an assumed name. Mrs. Pitezel tells me that the name her husband used in Philadelphia was B. F. Perry, which you will notice contains his own initials."

The insurance company discovered there was a policy for $10,000 on Pitezel's life and they announced that they would accept Perry as Pitezel if an independent person, other than a member of the family, would come forward and positively identify the body of Perry. They checked with the solicitor who told them, in passing, that Mrs. Pitezel had seen the news of her husband's death when it was reported in the Philadelphia local newspaper *Public Ledger*.

Consequently there arrived in the Friendly City a nice little man dressed in black, with a droopy walrus moustache and buckteeth, who announced in a chatty way that this was his first visit to Philadelphia and wasn't it sad that his first visit should be for such a doleful matter. He had with him a teenage girl named Alice who clutched at his hand and who he introduced as Alice Pitezel, the dead man's 15-year-old daughter. She had bravely volunteered to identify her father to satisfy the family that Perry was indeed Pitezel. The garrulous man gave his name as H. H. Holmes, said he was an inventor, just like his friend Perry, and mentioned that he had once employed Perry as a chemist in his Chicago drug store.

Alice was asked to look at her exhumed father and she identified him by the wide gap between his front teeth. After she left the room, Holmes took over. He said melancholy, "I fear it is my friend Pitezel. But to be sure, turn him over. You should find a wart at the back of his neck."

They did – and there was.

What Alice didn't know was that her father – strictly – shouldn't be dead. Holmes knew Pitezel was dead. He had killed him. Mrs. Pitezel, who was in on the plot, didn't think that the man being identified as her husband, was in fact actually him, for she believed him to be safely in hiding somewhere.

The plot was simple – or should have been. Pitezel (posing as Perry) was to open a laboratory in Philadelphia. After a time, Holmes was to arrive with a reasonably fresh corpse which roughly approximated Pitezel, and they would arrange the explosion. Pitezel would go into hiding, his wife would collect the insurance money and Holmes, being the accountant, would take it, count it, share it out.

Holmes, however, introduced his own wrinkle. He might have

tried to find a corpse like Pitezel, we'll give him the benefit of the doubt, but he soon discovered that Pitezel-shaped corpses were hard to come by. It might have been that while looking for one (wherever you look for corpses) the idea exploded in his mind that if Pitezel died he wouldn't need to lug a body all the way to Callowhill Street. Also, not to be over-looked, if Pitezel died he wouldn't need his share of the insurance. One idea led to another. If all the Pitezel family died, they wouldn't need money either.

Having carried through the first part of the scheme, Holmes had to do some crafty footwork as he put the second part into operation. Alice had seen her father's body and knew he was dead, so he had to keep Alice from any cosy chats with her mother. Alice had also talked to her sister and brother, so they had to be kept away from mother too. It was while he was busy taking care of them, and Mrs. Pitezel was waiting for the insurance money to arrive, that police detective Frank Geyer in Philadelphia put himself back on the case.

Probably the detective had been alerted by the insurance company. They had been asked to fork over $10,000 on a death which had, to say the least, several unusual features. They would have approached the police, in any case because of the nature of the death, in order to see if they had any doubts about it. They were gratified to learn that Geyer did; and Geyer was given a fresh charge of enthusiasm when he discovered that a false identity and a fortune was involved. While the Mutual Fidelity officials had been playing host to Holmes, they had been listening with great care to what the chatty man with the droopy walrus moustache and the weak eyes had to say.

They caught him out in a lie which wasn't really important but was worth remembering. Holmes had said that this was his first visit to the Friendly City but the carpenter, Eugene Smith, saw Holmes when the body was identified, and later told them that he had often seen Holmes visit Perry's laboratory.

Geyer was remembering what he thought was odd about the death scene in the laboratory. He couldn't be a hundred per cent sure about it, however, but he thought that if anybody was in an explosion in which their throat and lungs were seared, they wouldn't look as nonchalant as Perry had been in death. The inventor didn't actually have his hands casually in his pockets, but one had been draped across his chest, and the other hanging by his side. Geyer reasoned that anybody having his throat scorched by hot chemicals would raise his hands swiftly to his throat and neck. There had also been the unusual fact of the pipe, and that no glass shards had spattered the face of the man.

The insurance company came up with the information that the policy on Pitezel had *almost* expired. It was due to end on August 9. Then somebody had wired $157 50c. Less than a month later, on September 7, Pitezel was dead.

You could envisage the discussion in Holmes's Castle early in August, with conspirator Pitezel casually grumbling that he had a policy expiring and he hadn't had a cent on it. "Pity we can't find a way to milk it."

"Let me think about it, friend," Holmes would have replied. "If I can think of a way to make it pay for us, I'll pay the premium that's due."

"Give it some thought," Pitezel might well have replied. "It'd be a shame to waste it."

"Dear," Holmes might have said, turning to Minnie Williams, for she had been Queen of the Castle in August, "fresh cocktails all round." Then the mastermind had sat down to think about it.

Frank Geyer legged across Philadelphia and was pleased to discover that the stuff taken to the police scientific department from the Perry laboratory was still being held. He enlisted the help of the technicians. They carried out tests. They discovered that the glass vessel which was supposed to have exploded in Perry's laboratory held all its broken glass inside. Yet if a glass vessel explodes because its contents blow up, all the glass is showered outwards, not sucked inwards. On a similar vessel containing explosive materials they re-created the situation. The tests showed that the vessel from the laboratory had to have been empty at the time of the explosion.

The insurance company enlisted the help of the Pinkerton Detective Agency in Chicago and Geyer contacted other police forces. A call was made on Holmes Castle, but the doctor was gone. Nothing very suspicious in this for he had sublet his castle, which pointed against hurried flight. Penny-pinching Holmes hadn't wanted to miss a buck while he was away from home dealing with the Pitezel family. The detectives also looked for Jeptha D. Howe, the solicitor who had written the letter to the insurance company, and found him missing from his office, mysteriously vanished.

The Chicago police did know Holmes. Once some oil soaked rags had been found on some company premises, of which he was one of the directors.

The company didn't look too successful and they had checked out the directors. Nothing. Although the police suspected that arson was about to be carried out, they couldn't prove it, and the matter was forgotten. Geyer and other detectives now studied the director's list. The names were: A. S. Yates; Hiram S. Campbell; H. H. Holmes; Hermann W. Mudgett; Henry Owens; M. R. Williams.

The police themselves now began to check out the list. Mudgett was of course Holmes, but they hadn't discovered this yet. The only director they did find was Henry Owens, who turned out to be the porter whom Holmes had once nearly strangled. Owens didn't know who the other directors were, had never attended a director's meeting, and didn't even know that he had been an executive all this time. He gave it as his studied opinion that M. R. Williams was probably Minnie Williams, who had been the doctor's mistress. The authorities, without knowing she was dead, began tracking her back all the way to Texas. Meanwhile pieces of her body were in the cellar and her bones were on display in an anonymous medical school somewhere.

"There's a lot of mud around this Mudgett character," it was reported at a conference one morning. "About ten years ago he was studying medicine at the University of Michigan, and there were stories. A student friend died mysteriously and Mudgett picked up the insurance."

Detectives started to investigate the man without knowing he was Holmes. They found the insurance records too, showing that Mudgett had indeed collected $5,000 on the death of his fellow student. What kind of man, police began to wonder, insured his classmates? Or, putting it another way, what kind of company took that kind of insurance?

Mudgett was back-tracked to his home town of Gilmanton, New Hampshire. The detectives heard only good about him there. Holmes had had too much respect for Gilmanton to litter the place with corpses. But they discovered something else; only a few days before, the doctor had been seen around the town.

Meanwhile the Pinkerton detectives had reached Fort Worth, Texas, and discovered that M. R. Williams was, in fact, Minnie Williams. "No, Minnie wasn't there," said her friends. She had gone to Chicago a long time before to marry a doctor. Her sister had followed her and between them the girls had sold property in Texas valued at some $20,000. The Pinkertons were puzzled. Neither of the Williams girls had written home, they had not even sent cards at Christmas to their friends.

A Fort Worth bank had handled the sale of the property and a Chicago lawyer, they were told, had come to pick up the cash. His name was Benton T. Lyman. The Pinkertons produced photographs and Lyman was identified as Pitezel, alias Perry. The Detectives weren't long in Gilmanton before they discovered, by the descriptions they were given, that Mudgett was Holmes.

There just couldn't be two characters with droopy walrus moustaches, bad eyesight and buck-teeth roaming about. Things began to look clearer – Lyman was Perry who was also Pitezel; Holmes was Mudgett. What added to the confusion, apart from having several names, was that Pitezel and Holmes seemed to have had a lot of fancy professions. The neighbours in Chicago nearly came to fisticuffs arguing over what Holmes-Mudgett really did to earn his daily bread. Apparently, he had told something different to each of them. He was certainly a doctor, but at times, he had also claimed to be an inventor, estate agent, and chemist, but never a lady-killer. To clarify the position about Pitezel, his remains were dug up once more and his dentist finally identified him by his dental work.

Detectives were now hunting Holmes across several states. They traced him to Burlington, Vermont, and although they just missed him, they did discover that he had visited a woman who was staying in a bungalow with two young children. They called round and met Mrs. Pitezel.

Poor Mrs. Pitezel, who didn't yet know that her husband was dead, and that three of her children were soon to be murdered, admitted that there had been a plot. Holmes had visited her just recently, told her something had gone wrong and that her husband, Ben, was in hiding. She was asked where her three older children, Alice, Howard and Nellie, were and she said they were staying with a friend of the doctor's in Kentucky. Frank Geyer went looking for them on the half-mistaken theory that where the children were, Holmes might be. He went to Detroit eventually, after finding nobody in Kentucky, following a letter Alice had sent her grandparents. The scent led him from there to Toronto in Canada. He discovered that Holmes had arrived there but with only two children. The boy Howard was missing. Geyer began to get the shivers. He really began to shake when, aided by Canadian police, it was discovered that Holmes had left to return to the States and that when he left he was alone.

Holmes was tracked back to a hired, furnished bungalow. There a neighbour remembered him and the children, and also the fact that the friendly little man had asked to borrow a spade. In the cellar the police found Nellie's toy snake and, under the earth, the bodies of two girls. Holmes was moving fast, and by jettisoning the children, was able to move faster. Before going to Canada, he had rented a house in Indianapolis, and Howard's grave was found in the garden there.

Holmes had been hogging the headlines already but they became bigger with the news that three of the children had been murdered. Why Holmes felt compelled to murder them has never been satisfactorily explained. If he thought that they might give him away, he could easily have jettisoned them in a large city; leaving them at a railway station or even in a hotel, which would have given him ample time to escape. Since they were hardly in the plot, they wouldn't have been in for a share of the insurance loot in any case. And what plans did he have for Mrs. Pitezel and the two younger children? Had he planned to kill them but been thwarted because the police got to them first?

Holmes had another name by now – A. C. Hayes of Chicago. He was eventually arrested under this name in Boston, when he booked into a hotel there. Geyer arrived in time for the interrogation. Calm, yet weak and flabby looking, the little man in black showed his buck-teeth in a sardonic smile as he said: "Murder? Nonsesne. It was just an insurance swindle, pure and simple. I used a cadaver I procured from a New York morgue."

"Okay, then where is Pitezel?"

Holmes implied the question was stupid, for if they had the wife they should surely know. "Why, he's safely in South America of course"

Meantime, detectives were trying to trace other girls who had gone missing; those like Amelia Cigrand, Julia and Gertie Conner, Julia's child, Emeline Van Tassell, the Williams sisters, Mrs. Holden, and many others.

Holmes's Castle had been invaded and police were tearing it apart. The padded cells, peepholes, chutes and vats were found. A pit of quicklime also held secrets, notably the skeleton of a child, (presumed to be Julia Conner's eight-year-old daughter). Bits of bone, teeth, pieces of shoes, clothing and a gold watch, later identified as Julia's were found.

Holmes, making himself comfortable at police headquarters and behaving pompously, as was his customary manner, declined to admit that anything (other than a little high-spirited adventure to take the insurance company for a bundle) had occurred. Murder was beyond him – he was a simple, kindly man, and insurance companies deserved to be cheated. The missing girls? He was just as puzzled about their disappearance as anybody else. The dead Pitezel children – sad, but nothing to do with him. Finally he admitted that Perry had really been Pitezel. He maintained however, that Pitezel, a close friend, had committed suicide while in a deep melancholia from which even he was powerless to shake him. He stated:

"I came to Philadelphia and rented rooms at 1905 North Eleventh Street. Three days later Pitezel took the house at 1316 Callowhill Street, which he furnished partially with chemicals and bottles to represent a patent dealer. I visited the house, I think, four times besides the day on which he died. I visited the house the last of August and stayed five or six hours. At that time Pitezel was despondent. I found he had been drinking and took him to task for it. He remarked that he guessed he had better drink enough to kill himself and have done with it."

Benjamin Pitezel died on Sunday, and Holmes described the event as following:

"I went upstairs and laid down on the cot and read the paper. That was about twelve o'clock. After reading the paper for a half-hour I went to his desk to write some letters and found there a scrap of paper with a figure cipher on it that we used, and it said, 'Get letter out of cupboard.' I got the letter and it told me that he was going to end it all, and that I should find him upstairs if he could manage to kill himself. I ran up to the third storey and saw him lying on the floor dead. There was a towel over his face and a tube running from a bottle of chloroform."

Possibly the only truth was that Pitezel had been drinking and Holmes, a prude on alcohol, had criticized him. Smirking ingraciatingly and looking like a boneless toad, Holmes even attempted to make himself out as a hero. He had only rigged the suicide in an attempt to make it look like accidental death so that the widow and the children would get the insurance, which wouldn't be paid on self-destruction. Yes, Holmes would admit that it was fortunate in a way for him for Pitezel to be dead; it saved him the trouble, expense and danger of finding a cadaver who looked like him.

Holmes's pose throughout his arrest and trial was one of injured innocence, and he played it to the full and, a born actor, with some conviction. But the evidence against him was damning. We know little or nothing about his character, for it seems, shocked and horrified, his contemporaries wished to forget about him once he was executed. In the end he even tried to save his life by pleading insanity. He claimed, backing it with medical jargon, that he was suffering from a bone disease, which had affected both his mind and his body. The disease, he said, had elongated his head and made him resemble the devil. There were no psychiatrists attached to the American courts in 1894, so Holmes was never examined. It appears that Holmes liked to hide himself from the world, hence the castle, and was determined at all costs, to keep up a facade of respectability. His many mistresses were ostensibly in the building as secretaries, and when the porter Owens caught him making love to one, it sent him berserk.

Indeed, in his outwardly behaviour Holmes seemed to reflect much of the overbearing prudery of the times, a veritable Comstock. The marvel is that he kept his reputation intact among his neighbours around the castle when, in those days to be a bachelor and have two pillows on one's bed was to have one's reputation tarnished. His power over women was the most astonishing thing about him. Even when they discovered he was unfaithful to them they continued to stay with him under the principle, it seems, that half a loaf is better than none. They not only gave themselves, but as with the Williams sisters, their fortunes. Moreover, Holmes had not only the power of personality to win these women, but to comfort and reassure relatives and friends who must have come looking for them after they disappeared.

Holmes, with a guiltless expression, maintained his innocence throughout his trial, which opened in the Philadelphia City Hall on October 28, 1895. It lasted for six days. He had also maintained it through the earlier questioning about the murders of the three Pitezel children when detectives had re-placed him at the scene of the crimes. Throughout the trial he kept his cool and even managed at times to show a gallows sense of humour. When the jury left to consider the verdict, Holmes produced a coin from his pocket and tossed it." Heads not guilty – tails guilty," he said. To be sure, he tossed the coin ten times and nine times it came down heads – not guilty. The coin was wrong. He was found guilty and sentenced to hang.

He was determined to claim his innocence to the end, but a newspaper came up with a fat fee for his memoirs and greed, paramount in his make-up, won. He wrote a lurid confession in which he listed twenty-seven murders he had commttied. After he received the fee however, he denied that the confession was true. "I made it all up because I thought the paper should have its moneysworth," he said.

It was almost as if Holmes was two people – Holmes and Mudgett – and one person refused to believe what the other had done. On the gallows on May 7, 1896, just a week before his thirty-sixth birthday, Holmes did indeed make some sort of confession. He agreed that he had killed Emily Cigrand and Julia Conner – but hastened to add that they had died only after he had carried out abortions on them. Frank Geyer, who watched the hanging, left the prison a disappointed man. He had hoped Holmes would fill in the many gaps in his criminal career that the authorities had been unable to prove. But the little doctor in black, with the weak eyes, buck-teeth and walrus moustache swung from the world as if a martyr. As if he had been more sinned against than sinning.

DR. PHILLIP CROSS

The scene this bright June day could have stepped straight from a historical novel of the romantic variety, with not the merest whisper of Gothic horror. The high-stepping pony, the fast moving two-wheeled trap, and the pretty girl, holding on to her basket case with one hand and ensuring her bonnet remained in place with the other, who was staring ahead along the leafy lane for first sight of Shandy Hall, where she was taking up her new post as governess.

The date was June 1886, the place Dipsey, County Cork, Ireland, and the girl, Miss Mary Skinner, was joining the family of Dr. Phillip Cross as governess to the four Cross children at Shandy Hall. The twenty-year-old girl was all excited at the prospect of living among the county gentry.

Dr. Cross unfortunately, didn't have a successful practice in the district. It was unfortunate because, had he had a thriving practice, it might well have kept him out of mischief. He was tall and heavily bearded in keeping with the current fashion. He was sixty-two when the pretty governess came speeding through the gates of the estate, so he should have known better. Dr. Cross was "Indian Army Retired" and would moon about his estate most of the day, with nobody apart from his wife and four children and the servants to talk too. He looked into the distance as if he were once again accompanying columns of Redcoats across parched mountainous country in campaigns against fierce border raiders.

Dr. Cross may have been sixty-two but he felt thirty-two and Mrs. Cross, gathering the four squealing children in her wide embrace, would tell friends that: "Phil has the stamina and physique of a young man." She too thought it tragic that regulations had forced retirement on her husband at sixty and had sent them from the glamour and dangers of India to the regularity and solitude of County Cork.

Dr. Cross didn't complain because it wasn't the manly thing to do. "Damnit, only women and that sort of thing sit about and moan, what." But it must have seemed that the transition from the baked plains of India and an almost entirely masculine world to domesticity in County Cork, with rain and fog and screaming children, had been too swift, and the old doctor hadn't quite recovered his equilbrium yet. Mrs. Cross didn't help much. She, of course, missed the bustling, organised, chatty world of officers wives, where everybody, under the auspices of the colonel's wife, enthusiastically mucked in to make their corner of India home away from home.

A Victorian virtue decreed that the able bodied should work. Dr. Cross, even though retired from the army, carried on a practice of a sorts in the neighbourhood.

If later gossip is to be believed, and some of it should be, Dr. Cross didn't take too readily to hum-drum community practice. Colds and sneezes, cuts and bruises, were a far cry from the lopping of limbs and the grooving out of bullets following some bloody border battle. Mrs. Cross has been described as a colourless and drab woman. She was a quarter of a century younger than her husband, and the change in their environment had left her somewhat breathless, although she had the children and soon made friends in the district.

Dr. Cross, however, made few friends. The man who had once hunted tigers thought it ridiculous to chase the lowly fox, and he found he had little in common with the county gentlemen. This then was the circumstances at Shandy Hall, when the sprightly pony sped through the gates and carried Mary Skinner, her hair flying in the wind, up to the house and deposited her on the porch.

We know little of Mary (Effie was her nickname), apart from the gossip. One pressumes that she was from a genteel but impoverished family, perhaps even an orphan, and was forced to make her own way in the world until some gentleman asked for her hand. Unable to live by her own means, yet too good to be a servant, she had taken the compromise step which placed her halfway between the two as a governess.

Effie read a lot, more than was good for her, some would say with the confidence of hindsight, after the scandal had broken in the peaceful community. She read romances, the heavily melodramatic love novels of the times, in which the impossible all too frequently happened. Effie was said to be a day-dreamer and visualised herself as some sort of heroine. And here was the doctor, suntanned, fresh from the mysterious east, his taciturnity and long silences indicating a brilliant and reflecting mind at work.

Effie had been governess to the Caulfields, also a family of gentility, so she had not the merest gossamer whiff of scandal to blemish her name when the trap raced her to Shandy Hall. It is

quite possible, nobody can say for sure, that she might already
have set her frank blue eyes on the tall silent doctor, who looked
so like Abe Lincoln, before she even reached Shandy Hall,
maybe at some rustic frolic or other. Mrs. Cross certainly liked
Effie, as everybody did *before* it happened. People who once
couldn't find a bad thing to say about Effie, no matter how hard
they tried, couldn't find a good thing to say afterwards. But it
appears that she was both attractive and good humoured
(essential qualities for those who served) and we can only
imagine what effect she had on the introspected and introverted
doctor. We don't know how the affair started, and how, when it
did, they managed to keep it secret in a house with four scurrying
children and four or five hurrying servants. We can only visualise
the finger-licking circumstances. Was it a slow warm-up, beginning say with sly glances, and looks that became more ex-
pressively bolder with the passing of time and which eventually
became touches then grips? Or did the doctor, as is said to have
been usual in those times between master and servant, grab
Effie with hardly a word said and seduce her? Despite the doctor's
laconic manner, I prefer to believe the former.

But certainly it happened. We don't know how long it was
going on before Mrs. Cross stumbled over the lurid truth and,
ere the long hot summer had turned to winter, sent Effie thunder-
ing from Shandy Hall; ordered from house, town and even
county and refused a reference, without which important
missive she would be denied a like post and would be at the mercy
of the gutter.

The lovers, however, seemed to have had sufficient time to say
goodbye and make plans. Mrs. Cross, after all, wasn't all powerful even though right was on her side. Effie was ordered to go to
Dublin by Dr. Cross, there to await his coming. She seemed to
have sufficient funds to keep her from resorting to menial work
through the winter months. Dr. Cross couldn't rush to her until
the new year, leaving a lapse of time to allay his wife's suspicions.
After a few days with Effie in Dublin, the doctor returned to
Shandy Hall for a further interval, then started to visit Dublin
regularly and for extended periods. He told his wife it was
business interests and she, a dutiful Victorian wife, didn't
question when the doctor seemed declined to be more specific
or to elaborate.

By now Cross was certain he wanted to be with Effie permanently, and begrudged diluting his time with periods at
Shandy Hall. Divorce was difficult and if he lived openly with
Effie there would be disgrace. Much better therefore, he decided,
to keep his respectability by murdering his wife.

Mrs. Cross wasn't making too much noise about her husband's long absences in far off Dublin, and if she had any misgivings about them, she certainly kept loyal to her family and didn't mention the matter to her many friends.

But by now she had another problem. Her health was concerning her. Towards the end of January she became subjected to attacks of vomiting and diarrhoea. She also developed a burning thirst. Soon she was confiding bravely to her friends, "Phil is troubled. He doesn't think I'll last the year. He says I have a diseased heart."

Dr. Cross, talkative for once, (and people noticed his newfound friendliness), was also referring to his wife's repeated illnesses. Over the next five months, before she surrendered her life, Mrs. Cross's health went up and down like a yoyo. The doctor, still whistling to Dublin and back, told neighbours that the end was very near. Spring came. Mrs. Cross felt better. She began to hope and Dr. Cross, wiping away a tear, reassured her that she was on the mend. Then, a day or so later, he recharged her medicine with arsenic and strychnine – he was giving her both – and she was gravely and painfully ill again.

Those who had witnessed the doctor's diligence and affection in the care he gave his stricken wife, were to be horrified to the point of speechlessness with the revelation of the truth. They never imagined a person could be so callous, so hypocritical. Dr. Cross sought a second opinion by calling in his cousin, a Dr. Godfrey.

Dr. Godfrey, who was twenty-four, and just beginning his career, was impressed by his cousin's medical qualifications and military background and he looked upon him as the family's patriarch.

"It's typhoid fever of course, cousin," said Cross before Godfrey had seen the patient. Godfrey nodded, inspected the patient, and confirmed Cross's findings before leaving. The local parson also popped in but Cross reported his wife sleeping, and he had to be satisfied in joining the children in a moment of prayer.

It happened just a week later. A serving girl, Mary Buckley, was awakened by screaming. Superstitious, the frightened girl reacted by burying her head under the blankets. Shortly afterwards a tap came on the door and Dr. Cross said calmly, "Mary, get up. I want some help. Your mistress is dead." She found her master military brisk in manner and movements, and calm. In best army tradition, it seemed he was keeping his sorrow from the servants. Dr. Cross displayed a brutal and economical efficiency in all that followed. Mrs. Cross died in the early hours of the 2nd of June, and was buried in such a mean and hurried manner two mornings later, that it resulted in the gossip which would lead to the doctor's own disgrace and death. Dr. Cross ordered his wife buried at six o'clock in the morning. He gave her, at five pounds, the cheapest burial possible, which had the undertaker complaining that he had never seen anything like it from the gentry. Because of the early hour and because he had neglected to inform her many friends, nobody came to the funeral. Friends and relatives turned up later in the day, not sure of the time, puzzled by the hurry, and were shocked to find it all over.

There were one or two explanations, not very convincing. It was said that the doctor was used to Indian funerals. Burials took place there before the sun was up. But damnit all, this was Ireland, not India. People began to talk – not that Dr. Cross was around to listen. He spent several days tidying up and arranging for somebody to look after the children, and then left for England, arriving with Effie in London on the 9th, seven days after his wife's demise. If Dr. Cross had buried his wife with indecent haste, the neighbours in Cork had further shocks coming. Without waiting the prescribed six months or so, he remarried in even more indecent haste, in less than two weeks after his wife's death and, additionally, in the most flagrantly flashy manner he could think of.

One marvels at the doctor's stupidity and his arrogance astonishes. Having cunningly prepared the way for his wife and then brutally murdered her, one is surprised he didn't display the same slyness in regards to Effie. If he had to marry her right away, and she wasn't in a condition that he had to, he could have choosen an out of the way church or district in England. But not the besotted Dr. Cross. No. Nothing was too good for Effie. Dr. Cross married her at St James's Church, Piccadilly, in the heart of London, and the story got reported in all the society columns in the newspapers. Dipsey's entire population were reported to be flabbergasted. Was this an Indian custom too, dictated by the heat, they asked sardonically? There were other aspects of the affair to pull at. Apart from everything else, he had married somebody young enough to be his grand daughter, moreover somebody who had been in his employment but who had left rather suddenly and without any explanation. People just didn't leave jobs that quickly, nor that secretively.

There were still one or two lone voices speaking on the doctor's behalf. He was a soldier and they tended to be impatient and not know the right form. Moreover, he was getting on, didn't have a lot of time left, and presumably wanted to make the most of what he had. A well-wisher, however, decided to write to the doctor and acquaint him with a few home-truths.

A fashionable wedding was followed by fashionable parties, the best restaurants and hotels, and Effie must have thought it was a novel for her – a romantic novel – all come true. As she had driven up to Shandy Hall on that lovely summer's day she could never have dreamt that all this would follow within a year. Then the doctor received the letter from the well-wisher. He decided that the only way to stop the malicious gossip was to hasten back to Shandy Hall. Face the enemy squarely and frighten them, he decided, a good army tactic. Moreover, he must have reasoned, if Effie immediately took charge of the children (of whom she had been fond and they of her), people might begin to think, with a little encouragement from him, that he had really only hurried to remarry out of consideration for the children, poor motherless orphans who needed a motherly hand. Once installed in Shandy Hall, with all the dilution of entertainment that that implied. nobody could say they were having a high old time in the fleshpots of London.

The doctor announced their impending departure.

"Do we have to dearest?" asked Effie. It was almost as if she could now imagine the unhappiness which was to follow.

"Duty to my practice and the children calls, me-dear," he reprimanded.

On June 21, less than three weeks after he had buried his first wife, Dr. Cross was back in Shandy Hall with a more cuddlesome, baby-faced second one.

The couple received no welcome until they reached Shandy Hall, and then only from the children and the servants, who were duty bound by love or pay to smile. Effie must have soon been conscious of the ugly stares she received in the town and if the doctor never had a patient in his surgery, he still went there as if nothing untoward was happening. The doctor's behaviour had replaced the English as a subject for discussion and condemnation.

Dr. Cross must have decided that if he ignored it, the gossip would eventually die to be resurrected (only) from time to time over the tea cups and the Guinness. This might well have happened if an Inspector Tyacke of the Royal Irish Constabulary hadn't heard the rumours. When he began to check them, Tyacke was surprised to discover, as so rarely happened, that the rumours took on the deeper hues of facts. It really looked as if an old doctor had buried his wife in indecent haste after a mysterious illness, and then run off with a slip of a girl to London and there married her after only a few days. Well, well, well.

Tyacke called on the Coroner.

"Who did the p.m., then, on Mrs. Cross?"

"There weren't one."

"Why not?"

"Because a medical gentleman signed the death ticket."

"Which gentleman?"

"Why, the good husband, Dr. Cross himself."

"You'll see me here again."

"I'll look forward to the pleasure, to be sure."

Over the next few days the inspector could be seen strolling about the little town, smiling here, exchanging a word or two there, sipping a pint, making friends, and mollifying those who are traditionally wary of strangers. When they heard he was against Dr. Cross, they welcomed him quickly enough. He soon discovered the lie of the land and approached those who had genuinely known the Cross family and had something worthwhile to say. The Caulfield family, for whom Effie had once worked, were most helpful, and it was not only out of spite because she had left them as humble governess and was now mistress of Shandy Hall.

They were of the opinion that Mrs. Cross had sent Effie away after she discovered the girl and the doctor making love, and, certain that Dr. Cross had murdered his wife, they urged the inspector to have an exhumation made.

Inspector Tyacke didn't really have a lot to go on, just suspicion and the doctor's display of insensitivity and bad taste, but he deemed it sufficient to call on a local magistrate and demand an exhumation. It was an order that the magistrate, at first, was reluctant to give because Dr. Cross did have some standing in the district, and Tyacke's request was not backed by much evidence.

Eventually Tyacke got a hearing for his request. Even Dr. Cross turned up. He displayed a correct amount of repugnance and a restrained anger at the proceedings and the invasion of his wife's grave but refused to speak. The inquest was adjourned while a pathologist examined Mrs. Cross's remains. He found strychnine and more than three grains of arsenic in her stomach, proof that she had slowly been poisoned over a period of several months. The doctor was arrested at Shandy Hall the night before the inquest re-opened.

He was heard to say just after he was arrested to his sister, Henrietta, who lived at the Hall, "Did you destroy those two bottles with the white powder in them?"

The bottles were never found. Nor was any sign of a weak heart in Mrs. Cross, the ailment her husband had told her, would slowly kill her.

If the doctor kept up a military bearing outside the hall, Effie saw another side of him during those last few days before he was arrested. She didn't know exactly what was going on, but she

she saw her husband fade away overnight. The laughter left him. Suddenly he was his age. He hardly spoke to her or the children, and he locked himself away during those days while the remains of his first wife were being examined.

Until he met Effie Dr. Cross hadn't known the meaning of love. The first Mrs. Cross had been a nice woman, but he had never loved her. He had married her because it was the thing to do. In India, of course, there hadn't been much choice and he had never known many women. Then Effie had entered his life and it was like something he had never experienced before or even imagined; something he might have read in a book but simply didn't believe and dismissed as bunk. Dr. Cross had done a hateful thing, committed murder for love, and he must pay the penalty for it. Even though the incriminating medical bottles had vanished, the authorities had no great difficulty in pressing home their case against the doctor. The court, perhaps, wasted an unnecessary amount of time in establishing that Effie and the doctor had committed adultery in Dublin on diverse occasions and had lived together as Mr. and Mrs. Osborne. But they did establish that he had brought quantities of arsenic in Dublin and had told the chemist he wanted them for sheep dip.

After he was found guilty by the jury, Dr. Cross started an argument with the judge, attempting to explain why he couldn't be held responsible for the arsenic in his wife's stomach. The judge, a Murphy, refused to debate the matter, and sentenced him to death. After this, the doctor kept silent counsel. Perhaps he realised that had he shown the people of Dipsey a little more kindness, and had he spent a little more on the funeral, inviting the mourners to it at a respectable hour, he would have gone free and undetected. Again, if he had followed this by a less showy wedding, or even had waited six-months, he would well have been looked upon as a shining example of Victorian virtue in the community. A little more cool in the head and less heat in the blood would have left him laughing, instead of dangling from a rope on a chill January morning.

DR. THOMAS NEILL CREAM

If Thomas Neill Cream isn't the weirdest of the medical men in this collection, he is certainly the most colourful and, perhaps, the most mysterious. Before he went into the dim gas-lit streets of cities in England (and probably America and Canada) to carry out murder, he always dressed with care. This most fastidious of murderers would don a silk top hat, a velvet cloak over evening clothes, and sport a carnation and a gold-top walking stick. Nobody can be sure how many people Dr. Cream killed with his poisoned pills – invariably made up to look like sweets – because he didn't confess before his execution in London in 1892, and his brand of remote-control sadism – if it was sadism – is unique in criminal history, for he never waited to watch the death agony of his victims.

Another feature of Cream's crimes, which suggested there was a touch of conscience in him somewhere, was the often childish way he tried to attract the attention of the police to himself, often telling them that a victim had been murdered when foul play hadn't been suspected.

In the final stages of his career, when he was preying on the street girls in the less salubrious streets of London, Dr. Cream had fallen under the mesmeric spell of *Dr. Jekyll and Mr. Hyde*, the best selling novel of the time. There was another connection between the book's author, Robert Louis Stevenson, and Cream. Both had been born in Scotland in the same year – 1850.

The Stevenson novel – you will recall – told the tragic story of a gifted and eminent Harley Street doctor named Jekyll who plays with fire – the fire in this instance being powerful personality-changing poisons. The drug, Jekyll believes, can make bad men good, and he carries out experiments on himself. But as Jekyll is already a good man, it has a reverse effect upon him, neutralises his conscience and sense of duty and releases all the forces of evil in his sub-conscience. Thus, while under the influence, quiet Dr. Jekyll becomes the maniacal Mr. Hyde and dressed like a toff out-on-the-town in evening clothes – top silk hat and cloak and walking stick – terrorises those meaner beauties of the night in the more sordid thoroughfares of London.

The book hit Cream like a bomb. He raved to everybody about it. Not only did Cream identify with the hero, but also with the villain. After all, by day he was a hard-working, some even said gifted, medical practitioner; only he knew how he liked to wallow after dark in the illicit pleasures to be found in any large city. Cream was soon playing Mr. Hyde, prowling the gas-lit streets, jaunty of step, velvet cloak flying around his shoulders, gold-tipped stick swirling, hurrying to sauce-up the girls who loitered in dark doorways and passageways to offer loiterers tarnished love.

Cream had another characteristic, which, with his Phantom of the Opera apparel, made the sisters of sin remember him. He had eyes that suddenly moved into a cross-eyed position whenever he became excited. In impolite parlance, Cream was cross-eyed. But the eye-forking only happened after Cream had been indulging either in pleasures of the flesh, had been emotionally aroused, or lost his temper. It was a trait that helped bring him to the gallows.

But Robert Louis Stevenson cannot be held responsible for Creams' crimes, although he can be blamed – perhaps praised – for influencing the mode of dress Cream finally adopted. I say praised, for the theatrical costume helped in Cream's conviction. Cream had been committing murder long before the publication of *Dr. Jekyll and Mr. Hyde*. He began skittling people soon after he grew out of his teens. Since he never confessed, nobody can be certain how many murders he committed in, first, Canada, and then in the United States and Great Britain. His motives were just as baffling. In the beginning financial consideration, plus the bonus extra of lust, played a part in the motivation, but in the last year of his murderous reign Dr. Cream was comparatively wealthy and murdering just for the joy of it.

If Stevenson's novel was an influence on Cream, so too were the crimes of Jack the Ripper. Although Cream was in an American prison finishing a sentence for murder when Jack the Ripper was terrorising Whitechapel, he would obviously have read about it and he arrived in London three years after the Ripper's last murder, so there would still have been discussions about it. Like the Ripper, Cream terrorised cheap prostitutes in the streets at night and he had a less messy, if more painful way of despatching them.

Cream was born in Glasgow in 1850, one of the children of a wealthy shipbuilder, who decided to emigrate to Canada when Cream was three years old. Cream was said to be of advanced intelligence and even though he was surrounded with brothers and sisters, he was considered a child recluse. A peculiarity

showed itself in him at an early age, for when he became angry
or excited his usually normally-spaced eyes would snap towards
each other and lock in a cross-eyed position until he had calmed
down. This became noticeable in his student days, especially
when he had been out with girls, and he came in for a lot of
risqué leg-pulling from fellow students because of it.

Cream eschewed sports and games and preferred, instead,
books and his own company. At the junior school in Quebec
he was known as either "Mr Encylopaedia" because of his learning, or "Mr Cyclops" because of the fault in his eyes. He
decided on medicine and went to McGill College, Montreal,
where a generous allowance from his father enabled him to
dress like a dandy. He wore jewellery and even kept a carriage
and pair and although very much the recluse still, he had the
reputation of being a rake.

But if Cream was raking hard in the gas-lit streets at night, he
was working hard at his books by day, and he often had to be
warned to take it easy for his eyes would also cross with fatigue.
Cream was deeply religious and found the time to preach to
children at a nearby church. Good and evil were close friends of
his, however, even then, for he produced a series of brilliant
essays on the effect drugs and poisons had on the body. While
full of praise for his efforts, the professors thought he was
showing an inordinate interest in toxicology and tried to divert
his attention to healthier things.

Cream graduated as an MD – with merit – in March 1876.
The dean of the faculty gave a graduation address on the evils
of malpractice in the medical profession, and Cream – who would
soon kill a girl in a botched backroom abortion – hurried to
congratulate him and agree with the noble sentiments expressed.

Cream was due to leave college and had no further use for the
furniture and fixtures in his room. By chance – he said – a fire
broke out and he claimed a thousand dollars insurance. But the
company checked the fire, found little of worth left in the room
and detected evidence of arson. But, rather than contest on
flimsy evidence they compromised by offering Cream 350 dollars.
Cream accepted. The graduate was also in trouble at Waterloo,
Quebec Province, where Eliza Brooks, with whom he had had an
affair, was seriously ill. It was discovered that Cream had given
her an abortion and Mr. Brooks told Cream that if he wouldn't
marry his daughter he would shoot him. Cream married Eliza.

Cream was so incensed at this shotgun trickery that he left
for England the day after the wedding, claiming it was imperative
he complete his medical studies there. He did this at St. Thomas's

Hospital, London, and in Edinburgh, and qualified both as surgeon and physician.

Just a year after he had arrived, he heard news from Canada that his wife was dead.

Cream now returned to Canada and started a practice in London, Ontario, but soon after a girl was found dead in the yard behind his surgery. It looked as if she had been dumped out with the rubbish. There was a bottle of choloroform beside her but it was established that she couldn't have taken this herself. At the inquest, it was also stated that she had been visiting Cream, who she knew well, to procure an abortion. Cream was called and said that the girl had come to him and accused a leading local merchant of seducing her. The merchant, denying this, produced documentary evidence to show that some sinister and mysterious person was trying to extort money from him by saying he had evidence that he had seduced the girl. It would seem that at this early stage in his career, Cream was writing mischievous and juvenile letters. Nothing could be proven, however, and a verdict that the girl had died by the hand of a person unknown, was given. But Cream as the chief suspect was ruined and decided next to try the wider pastures of the United States.

People had mixed views about Cream. They agreed he was brilliant and painstaking, but found him lacking in principle. He seemed always to be on the look out for abortion work, and not just because he was short of money. He got a kick out of doing something illegal and he liked the hold it gave him over a girl who had already shown herself willing.

Cream set up practice in Chicago and about now he discovered he had a strange and compelling hypnotic power in his eyes. He made the discovery when trying to cure a child of epileptic fits. After he had bounced the child on his lap for a time, she told her father that the doctor's eyes made her tingle all over and made her relax. Cream tested his hypnotic powers on other patients and found they worked. He was soon advertising cures by hypnotism and he was scrutinised by the American Medical Association for quackery, but they eventually ruled that although they couldn't explain his power he wasn't doing anything unethical. But Cream was soon in trouble in the windy city for abortion offences. A girl named Julia Faulkner died in 1880 after an illegal operation, and Cream was arrested. The case was dropped because of inconclusive evidence. Just four months later another girl died, this time from faulty drugs which Cream had supplied. Cream wrote blackmailing letters to the druggist, Frank Pyatt, saying he could prove he was responsible, and unless he paid up he would take the facts to the police. Pyatt was of the opinion that Cream had tampered with the drugs after they had left his store and he was right. Cream was doing the same thing in an effort to get rid of the husband of the girl he loved.

She was a beautiful natural blonde named Mabel Scott from Garden Prairie, a Chicago suburb. She had called with her husband Daniel, in answer to Cream's advertisement that he could cure fits by hypnotism. Danny was sixty and was suffering from attacks of sudden spasms – hardly conducive to his lot because he was a telegraphist with the Chicago and Northwestern Railway.

We don't know if Cream cured the involuntary shake in the telegraphist's hand, but we have ample evidence that he worked his wicked hypnotic will on Mabel. Cream found sufficient numbers of things wrong with Danny to keep Mabel coming to the surgery and they were soon sleeping together. Neighbours would testify at Cream's trial that he was often seen popping into the Scott household after Danny had left with his food box for the day, and he would stay there all night when Danny went on transcontinental journeys.

Soon Cream was telling Mabel how blissful it would be if they were together all the time, and Danny's medicine was soon being laced with strychnine. But since marriage, home and children, even in those days, called for great quantities of cash, the couple thought they would insure Danny's life so he could give them a good start when he was out of the way.

The couple worked hard to get Danny insured, forging his name to policies or inveigling him into signing them by claiming they were something else. Even though Cream had good connections in the medical and insurance fields, Danny's health was so bad that nobody would insure him. The couple finally decided he would have to go without leaving them a handsome wedding present and Danny received the dose that kills. Since Cream, as family doctor, signed the death certificate, there was no unhealthy interest shown in Danny's demise by the authorities.

The Garden Prairie neighbours were gossiping. Mabel got a shock when she suggested to one that she was hoping she might marry again in the not too distant future. Sniffing sourly, the neighbour said, "Not that crazy looking doctor with the funny eyes, I hope."

Local legend said that Cream was so incensed when Mabel told him this that he thought of topping up the woman's doorstep milk with strychnine. But there were no other problems, nor would there have been, had not Cream got one of his mad get-rich schemes going. He wrote to the Boone County Coroner that Scott had died because the chemist had mistakenly put too much strychnine in his medicine. His plan was to get Scott exhumed the poison found, and then have Mabel sue the chemist for a couple of hundred thousand dollars for negligence.

But the coroner decided to ignore Cream's complaint, because although it was from a doctor, he thought it was written probably in a hysterical and bombastic manner. Angry because authority wouldn't move in the matter, Cream rushed to see the district attorney and rudely demanded action. Cream got more action than he wanted. The police investigated Cream, and when they discovered that the doctor who had signed the death certificate had been having an affair with the wife and it now looked as if they would marry, they decided to exhume Scott. Four grains of strychnine were found, and Mabel Scott, to save herself, turned state's evidence. Cream, struck dumb by her treachery, stood trial alone, and was sentenced to life imprisonment for, surprisingly, murder in the second degree.

Cream took the sentence calmly. But he was most bitter about Mabel's defection and betrayal. It was the second time in his life, he confided to prison inmates, that he had been wronged by a woman. Although the girl who had tricked him into marrying her in Canada was now dead, Cream would often rage against her. And now – a second time – there was Mabel. During his term of imprisonment, Cream's dislike of the fair sex blossomed into a cold illogical hatred. There was an element of religious fanaticism in it. Hadn't they, with their lascivious ways, lured him away from God?

Cream worked hard at Joliet penitentiary, Illinois, and it was because of his medical and religious work among the inmates that he won a parole in July 1891 – after serving ten years.

He could little know, as he stepped through the iron gates to freedom, that imprisonment and execution by hanging, was only some eighteen months and three thousand miles or so away. But by his speed of movement it is obvious he left Joliet with a purpose and a plan. Cream's father had died five years before and left him sixteen thousand pounds so he didn't have the need to earn a living to encumber his movements. It is said, by one source, that he went straight to Garden Prairie to look for Mabel and to kill her. But, sensibly, she had vanished years before.

He spent only a few weeks in America. Then he took ship to England, where he landed on October 1.

By October 4, Cream was in London, and on the following night, dressed in his Phantom of the Opera costume, was making himself known to the street girls of London. Soon they would be talking among themselves about the tall "gent" with the Ameri-

can accent, the almost bald head and the heavy ginger moustache
– and, of course, the peculiar eyes. They found Cream's eyes
unusually bright and it caused them no end of amusement when
they saw how the eyes crossed when he was gripped with excite-
ment. Some of the girls maintained later that Cream was heavily
bearded, and it appears that at times he did don a costume piece
as a disguise.

On October 7, describing himself as a Dr. Neill, Cream moved
into lodgings at 103 Lambeth Palace Road. There were medical
students from St. Thomas's Hospital staying there and Cream
made himself known to them and was sentimental enough to
visit the old hospital where he had taken training more than
fifteen years before. Next morning he visited a chemist shop in
Parliament Street, told an assistant he was lecturing at the
hospital and asked for nux vomica – which contains strychnine.
As it was a scheduled poison he had to sign the book and give
his address. He signed "Thomas Neill, M.D.," and gave his
present lodgings.

What surprised the girls about "Toff Fred", as they called
him, was the elaborateness of his approach and the interest he
took in all aspects of their lives. Most of them were casual girls
who invariably knew their clients for only five or ten minutes;
they had no regulars, and knew nobody by name. But Cream
adopted the practise of stopping girls in the street to make
appointments for some time later in the week. This must have
surprised them.

"Guess what? I met a gent who wants me by appointment
only."

The girls took an interest in "Fred the Toff" because he took
an interest in them. It wasn't so much the jingling guineas and the
flashing jewellery on his fingers and shirt front, but the fact that
they saw in him a kindred spirit, another of life's rejects, another
lost soul and very far from home. What final irony, then, that
Cream was out to destroy them.

There must have been several thousand street girls in the Waterloo Bridge and Station area were Cream prowled before the turn
of the century. And very few people took an interest in them.
To be sure religious and charitable organisations would make
periodic raids – and the occasional religious zealot's interest
wasn't always of the purest motive. Sin was considered disgusting
and an interest in sex unhealthy, and clients invariably loitered
in dark alleyways with their coat collars up. So nobody wanted
to know them or talk to them after the business was done and a
few sweaty shillings changing hands.

None of the girls was missed when they died, as they frequently did from neglect, malnutrition or a crushed spirit in their sordid backrooms, and invariably they were found to be penny-less and property-less when the authorities arrived. No doctor looked too closely to determine cause of death before signing a death certificate, and they would be buried disinterestedly and cheaply in a pauper's grave paid for by the parish. Their real names, religions, and from whence they came, was rarely known.

And here was Cream paying them courteous court and taking more than a sexually superficial interest in them. No wonder they responded, even if, as some of them did, they found those weirdly-crossing eyes frightening and funny.

Cream told them he was a doctor. He was concerned about the way they neglected themselves. They should eat regularly and wear warmer clothing, He pressed pills upon them, to improve their health, he said, so why shouldn't they swallow them? Some of them did – almost the last action they made. It was so easy. But for the Dracula-like costume and those crossed eyes Cream could have gone on forever, for he ordered poisoned drugs by the hundreds. When his victims died in excruciating agony hours later they were invariably too ill to tell anybody about "Fred the Toff's" pills which they had taken, and the local doctor – who usually arrived after death had taken place – seeing that the corpse had been another impoverished prostitute, wouldn't find murder because he wasn't looking for it.

The street girls were in the capital in their thousands and we have no idea, so long after the events, how many girls he might have killed during his nightly forays over some eighteen months. He had the Whitechapel area in the east, Lambeth in the South, Paddington in the west, as well as the more fashionable areas of central London to prowl. He made a brief and mysterious return to the United States and Canada for about four months, where he purchased five hundred strychnine pills and nobody knows if he poisoned prostitutes while he was there also.

In London, a fortnight after his first arrival, a prostitute named Ellen Donworth, aged 19, was his first known victim. She was walking her beat in the Waterloo Road on the evening of October 13, when she collapsed to the road. Witnesses who went to help her said her face had turned as white as a sheet, that she was twitching uncontrollably and was convulsing in all her limbs. They took her into a house and it took several men to hold her down as she screamed and struggled like a lunatic. In the short intervals when her agony abated, she said, "A tall gentleman with cross-eyes, a silk hat and bushy whiskers gave me a drink twice out of a bottle . . . there was white stuff in it." She also said that she had known the man, had not just met him and, in fact, had received two letters from him, but, at his request, had given him back the letters when she met him at six that evening at the York Hotel in Waterloo Road. She had begun to feel ill an hour after she had left him.

Ellen Donworth died after reaching St. Thomas's Hospital, and an examination of her stomach revealed strychnine. The Coroner, GP Wyatt, received a letter through the post, which — for the time — was ignored.

The letter read:

> "I am writing to say that if you and your satellites fail to bring the murderer of Ellen Donworth, alias Ellen Linnell, late of 8 Duke Street, Westminster Bridge Road, to justice, that I am willing to give you such assistance as will bring the murderer to justice, provided your government is willing to pay me £300,000 for my services. No pay if not successful.
>
> A. O'Brien, Detective."

O'Brien showed intimate knowledge of the girl, her previous used name in particular, but if the authorities were now of the opinion that the young prostitute had been murdered, they weren't too enthusiastic about attempting to track down her killer. In the shifting world of casual acquaintanceship at the lower fringes of society, nobody knew much about his neighbour and what he did know he was reluctant to talk about. The police had enough to do already and their first concern must be the protection of the respectable and law-abiding members of society. They would put the Donworth file to one side and wait and see what developed. If the killer struck again, or if he turned his attention on the more deserving members of the public, then that would be the time to pull in the weights, flick the whips and get all available hansom cabs on the go. O'Brien did reveal intimate knowledge of the dead girl, but that didn't mean he was the murderer. And the reward he asked for showed him to be more crank than criminal.

Cream's next known victim was Matilda Clover, of 27 Lambeth Road. Matilda was seen with Cream a few days before he murdered her, which was only a day or two after Ellen Donworth died. There seemed to be a pattern in his crimes. He would see the girls on two or three occasions and eventually, as if tiring of them, slip them the pill. Elizabeth Masters saw Matilda and Cream meet — and it made her angry. She knew Cream herself, having met him a few days before, and in the post that day Elizabeth had got a letter from Cream saying he would be popping around that afternoon. Elizabeth was watching for him and as he turned the corner into Lambeth Road, she saw Matilda come from her house to solicit, and accost Cream.

Cream was interested immediately. He forgot about Elizabeth, who cursed and told a friend, and they watched the couple disappear. Elizabeth was miserable – then. But it was good fortune for Elizabeth, bad news for poacher Matilda.

On October 19, a scrubbing girl named Lucy Rose was cleaning out Matilda's furnished room when she saw a letter. Like serving girls will do, she took a moment off from her unrelenting drudgery and read the missive, which she assumed to be a love letter. She was a little disappointed for it was blunt and to the point and, if truthful, a downright embarrassment for Matilda. It said:

"Meet me outside the Canterbury (a famous music hall) at 7.30 if you can come clean and sober. Do you remember the night I bought you your boots? You were so drunk that you could not speak to me. Please bring this paper and envelope with you.

Yours,
Fred."

Lucy Rose hadn't seen Matilda leave the house so she didn't know if the girl, in obedience to Cream's paternal and scolding advice, had gone clean and sober and wearing the new boots he had bought for her, but later that night, when she opened the door for Matilda, the girl had an escort. Lucy Rose could see the gentleman because there was a small paraffin lamp in the hall. She said at Cream's trial that the "gentleman was tall and broad and had a heavy moustache. He was wearing a large coat with a cape on it, and a high silk hat."

Lucy Rose said that, having brought Matilda home the gentleman left, and she heard Matilda say to him "Good night, dear." Lucy Rose was awakened at three o'clock by screams from Matilda's room. She found Matilda lying across the foot of her bed with her head fixed between the bedstead and the wall. "She was apparently in great agony, and she told me she had been poisoned by pills given her by the gentleman," Lucy Rose testified.

Although a doctor was called, one didn't arrive until lunchtime on the following day, but an unqualified assistant had been sent during the night with medication. A Dr. Graham came at lunchtime but all he had to do was sign a death certificate because Matilda had died at nine that morning. Since Dr. Graham had been treating Matilda for alcoholic poisoning, he gave the cause of her death on the certificate as "primarily delirium tremens, secondly syncope."

Matilda was buried, and, for a time, forgotten, and a day or two after she died, Cream picked up another prostitute. This was away from his customary haunts in the more fashionable West End. The girl said her name was "Lou" Harvey, and that she lived with an artist, named Harvey, as his wife, in a studio in St. John's Wood. Cream took "Lou" to dinner and they spent the night together in a West End hotel. Over breakfast in the morning, Cream told the girl that she had some spots on her forehead and if she would meet him later he would give her some pills to remove them. When Lou got home she told her painter friend about Cream and the pills and said she found him odd but she thought she would go and meet him, that is if the friend thought it would be all right. Harvey thought it strange and suggested he go with her, and they saw Cream at the stated place on the embankment at eight o'clock on the following evening. The painter kept back while the girl approached Cream. She testified later: "He took two pills out of his waistcoat pocket. They were wrapped in tissue paper. He gave them to me and said I was to take them, and he said I was to put them in my mouth then and there, one by one, and not bite them but swallow them."

Lou said, "He put them into my right hand. I put my hand to my mouth and pretended to swallow them, but I passed them into my left hand. It was a good thing I did, for he asked me to show him my right hand to see if I had taken them. I showed him and it was empty. He then asked me to show my other hand, so I threw the pills away behind me and showed him my empty hand." Cream then bade Lou goodnight and offered to call her a cab, but she wanted to go to a music hall with him, as he originally suggested they would – hence the meeting – but he excused himself by saying something important had come up and he had to go to St Thomas's Hospital. He said, however, he would see her later, at eleven o'clock, but he didn't turn up. It was Cream's biggest mistake, for he assumed Lou had swallowed the pills and would be dead before the night was out.

There were already rumours among the street girls who were warning each other to avoid "a gent with crossed eyes and a ginger moustache who talks like a Yank and tries to get you to take capsules." But, judging by his behaviour with Lou Harvey, Cream hadn't curtailed his activities to let things quieten down, although he was, as he had done for Lou Harvey, going away from his usual haunts.

Some three weeks later Dr. William Broadbent, one of London's most distinguished physicians, received a letter in the post. It was signed by somebody called "M. Malone," and it stated:

"Sir,

Miss Clover, who, until a short time ago, lived at 27 Lambeth
Road, South London, died at the above address on October
20 (last month) through being poisoned with strychnine. After
her death a search of her effects was made, and evidence
was found which showed that you not only gave her the medicine which caused her death, but that you had been hired
for the purpose of poisoning her. The evidence is in the hands
of one of our detectives, who will give the evidence either to
you or to the police authorities for the sum of £2,500 sterling."

Dr. Broadbent couldn't remember when he had last been south
of the Strand, and since Mr Malone had not given an address,
he couldn't reply. But he placed the letter on one side for the
police, as did the Countess Russell who, while staying at
the Savoy Hotel, received a letter saying that her husband, the
Earl Russell, had murdered a prostitute named Matilda Clover
in Lambeth Road. The second letter in particular was to
damage Cream at his trial for nobody knew at the material
time that Matilda Clover had been poisoned. Of course,
Cream had made hardly any attempt to disguise his handwriting.
But not all Cream's social activities were restricted to nefarious
nocturnal pursuits around the more questionable London
haunts. Dressed in his best bib and tucker he had permission
from a Mrs Sabbatini to call at her home at Berkhampstead,
twenty miles from London, and pay his respects to her charming
daughter. The Sabbatini were genteel with social pretentions and
for Cream there could be no hankypanky there. These were short
and polite visits for tea, a walk in the gardens which gave Cream
a chance to demonstrate his abilities on the piano. Love bloomed
slowly in these visits which always ended before dark.

About the time Cream began popping pills into Lambeth's
poppet-aged prostitutes, he was also on his knees before Laura
Sabbatini at Berkhampstead, popping the important question
and promising her undying affection. She was honoured by his
offer of marriage and accepted it.

In January Cream went to America and Canada. He gave Laura
no particular reason for the trip, and none was forthcoming.
After his arrest the Sabbatinis moved discreetly from the picture
so what they knew wasn't made public.

We know that Cream was in the Blanchard's Hotel, Quebec,
for several nights. He met a commercial traveller named M'Culloch there who would never forget a peculiar conversation in
which Cream did all the talking. It had him studying the newspapers for many months, checking to see if any young girls had
been found poisoned to death in the streets.

Cream flashed a bottle at M'Culloch in the bar, and said, with pride, "See that? That's poison. Do you know what I do with it. I give it to women. Act? It acts faster than a stain remover. Whoof and they are dead."

Cream then produced small capsules of the sweetened jelly kind.

"See these, brother? I give it to them in these. Then they don't notice the taste, see."

Cream also produced from his pocket a pair of false whiskers, and he added, "When I'm operating I always wear these to prevent identification if there is a slip-up."

Cream was often indiscreet with strangers, an indiscretion that rivalled those he made in print. He always carried pornographic pictures on him and could be seen studying these in pubs, on trains and in other public places – and was ever ready to show them around. He also told drinking cronies that he was partial to drugs, especially those of an aphrodisiacal kind, and he claimed to suffer from migraine and insomnia.

He called on a Quebec City drug manufacturer and ordered five hundred strychnine tablets of a dosage which was definitely lethal. It is said the manufacturer didn't like Cream too much and declined an offer Cream made to act as the firm's European representative. But he accepted an order Cream gave for a further five hundred lethals.

Cream also called on a Quebec printer and had five hundred circulars printed, which said:

ELLEN DONWORTH'S DEATH:
TO THE GUESTS OF THE METROPOLE HOTEL   —
Ladies and Gentlemen,
I hereby notify you that the person who poisoned Ellen Donworth on 13th last October is today in the employ of the Metropole Hotel and that your lives are in danger as long as you remain in this Hotel.
Yours respectfully,
W. H. Murray.

London, April 1892

We don't know what the Canadian printer thought because he seems to have thought it not worthy of comment; nor do we know why Cream chose the Metropole Hotel of all hotels in London. The presumption is that he had a grudge because he was thrown out of the hotel bar. After three months on the loose in the Western Hemisphere, and doing what we can only imagine, Cream arrived back in London on April 9. He went to his lodgings at Lambeth Palace Road and just two nights later, went into action again. On April 12, a policeman named George Cumley saw a man being let out from a side door at 118 Stamford Street. It was a quarter to two in the morning. Cumley clearly saw the girl who waved the man goodbye.

Constable Cumley knew that two street girls lived in the house – Emma Shrivell, aged 18, and Alice Marsh, aged 21 – and it was Emma who let the gentleman out. The constable recognised him as a gentleman by his expensive cloak and silk top hat and he got a clear look at him as he danced beneath a gas lamp and heard him give off a fiendish laugh. Others had heard that laugh, but few had lived to talk about it. Lou Harvey had heard it on the Thames Embankment after surreptitiously discarding the pills Cream had given her. As he danced off into the night believing that she was but an hour or two away from death, she heard a maniacal laugh which sent ice-like shivers of fear down her spine.

Constable Crumley continued on his night beat and three-quarters of an hour later horrifying shrieks disturbed the stillness of the Victorian night. When the constable patrolled back that way again, all lights in the house were burning and there was much coming and going. Each of the girls had a room for which they paid 12/6d (62½p) per week, and it was from Alice's room that the screams first came. The landlady ran upstairs and found Alice huddled on the floor in an extremity of pain. A minute later there came screaming from Emma's room, and the landlady also found her writhing on the floor in agony. A policeman named Eversfield was brought to the house. He gave the girls emetics of mustard and water, then took them by cab to hospital; Alice died before they reached St. Thomas's Hospital, which was nearby, but Emma lingered on for six hours before expiring.

Emma managed, between bouts of fearful pain, to tell Crumley that she had entertained a toff named Fred. Fred had said he was a doctor. Alice, he and she had dined on tinned salmon and bottled beer and Fred had given each girl three long pills which, he claimed, would be beneficial. First medical appraisal was that the girls had died from strychnine.

Cream read about the inquest at his lodgings. It was Easter Sunday. We get a vivid picture of him pacing from the dining room to the sitting room in that neat, tidy, genteel Victorian boarding house for gentlefolk where everybody was respectfully addressed by title, where silence was the paramount characteristic.

We have courtroom testimony by the landlady's daughter, a Miss Sleaper, on how angry Cream became on reading the Sunday papers. Cream was in a rage, stomping the carpet.

"What cold-blooded murder, Miss Sleaper! What wicked

viciousness there is in the world. Something must be done to bring the fiend to justice and execution."

That was Cream in the drawing room as Miss Sleaper remembered him – and she was concerned because his loudness and the verocity of his manner might cause distress to other guests.

Another study of the paper, and Cream stopped her from her dusting again as, with determination, he shouted: "I fear the police are fools. I think I must conduct an investigation myself. Why, Miss Sleaper, I will not rest until I have brought the miscreant to justice."

Fifty years on, and Miss Sleaper's own maturing and a more sophisticated public taste might have made her decide Cream was ham acting, and a not very convincing ham at that. We cannot be sure what the gentle Miss Sleaper thought at the time.

Popular fiction had already began to feature the citizen as hero-detective, and Miss Sleaper must have thought that Dr. Neild – as she called him – sounded like somebody out of a "lurid penny-dreadful".

But it became lurid fiction with a sinister aspect a little later in the day when Cream happened to pass the room of another lodger, a William Harper. The door stood open and there was Miss Sleaper waving a duster like a magic wand. Harper, a medical student at St. Thomas's, was absent, and Cream lunged into the room and in a stage whisper told Miss Sleaper something which made her recoil with fright. Cream said that he suspected young Harper of the murder of the two girls, and urged her to tell him all she knew about the student.

Then Cream, apparently looking like Groucho Marx playing Sherlock Holmes, prowled the room glaring at things as if looking for incriminating clues. Miss Sleaper, already embarrassed by Cream's invasion of a room not his own, was further horrified to hear Cream become more emphatic that Harper was the murderer. Earlier she had excused it on the grounds of jealousy, but now she rounded on Cream. "Dr. Neild," she said, "I will not hear these vile accusations against Mr. Harper any more, if you please. They are in shocking taste, to say the least. You have no right in his room and I order you, forthwith, to withdraw from it."

Cream, who was not without manners, bowed and left.

Cream had already made himself known at nearby St. Thomas's Hospital as an old student. He drank with the doctors and students and talked about the "good old days" when he had studied there fifteen years before.

Legend even has it – though it sounds too good to be true – that Cream visited the mortuary when Ellen Donworth, his first known victim, was being examined. "Who is this?" he is supposed to have asked a surgeon. Told she was Donworth, the prostitute, and that her death was due to strychnine poison, Cream is alleged to have replied:

"Suicide, I imagine. Couldn't face her shame any longer. A pity, really, such a pretty lass."

Just as incredible – and this is established fact – was that descriptions of "Lord Fred" as the sensational press dubbed him, were appearing in the newspapers. The descriptions were so accurate that it is strange nobody saw the similarity and reported Cream to the police. The killer in the newspapers was reported to be balding, had ginger moustache, and claimed medical qualifications.

But Cream didn't leave the matter there. He would buttonhole doctors and students at the pubs near the hospital, and say, "They even say he has eyes that cross in some of the newspapers, and my eyes cross too."

"You should sue the chap for posing as you," would come the answer.

And Cream would reply, "Funny if you were drinking with the fiendish poisoner, eh?"

Cream's favourite suspect, young Harper, was the son of Dr. Joseph Harper of Barnstable, and a week after Easter the doctor received a letter from somebody signing himself "W. H. Murray" which said:

> "I am writing to inform you that one of my operators has indisputable evidence that your son, W. J. Harper, a medical student at St. Thomas's Hospital, poisoned two girls named Alice Marsh and Emma Shrivell, on the 12th inst. and that I am willing to give you the said evidence (so that you can suppress it) for the sum of £1,500 sterling. The evidence in my hands is strong enough to convict and hang your son, but I shall give it to you for £1,500 sterling or sell it to the police for the same amount."

Since Cream never attempted to follow up such letters and extort money – he wasn't short of cash in any case – there are all types of reason put forward why he wrote them. It is not enough to say that he was insane, for there had to be a motive. If Cream was insane – and some people would say that all murderers are mad – then the people who he socialised with, including eminent doctors, didn't think he was anything more than eccentric and a little extravagant when he became drunk or excited. It has been suggested that Cream, by now a living counterpart of Robert Louis Stevenson's Dr. Jekyll and Mr. Hyde, was ashamed of his atrocious crimes and was writing the letters, in a sense, to hasten his capture so that he could be prevented from committing further murders, which, in the cold light of morning, filled him with revulsion. Such actions by mentally-disturbed criminals are not, of course, rare, and Cream, remember, was deeply religious. He didn't don his Phantom of the Opera costume *every* night and seek victims in the murky gas-lit streets. Some evenings found him seated at the organ in the drawing room of the genteel boarding house, soothing the other guests with religious music, impeccably rendered. He also called regularly on his fiancée, Miss Sabbatini, although convention would demand that he stay there for only a few hours and return before bedtime.

And then again the letters could have been a cunning ploy on Cream's part, for assuming that his actions might eventually get him caught, he was publishing proof which pointed to insanity, and this would, he hoped, save him from the gallows. Or, on the other hand, perhaps it was all an exciting parlour game, a crime puzzle, a test, a competition, in which he sent clues winging away so that the police had something to go on and could begin to track him down. If he could make it more cat-and-mouse, for the police seemed to be baffled and bungling, then it would become that much more exciting.

But in planting these clues, Cream eventually went too far. After all, he had been dancing around the police all his life and literally getting away with murder. He had only come a cropper once – in the Scott affair – and that had been because a woman had betrayed him. But even then he had escaped execution. So, with arrogant confidence, Cream called on the police.

He talked to a Sergeant McIntyre, to whom he had been introduced by a mutual friend, and showed him a letter which had gone through the post and was addressed to the dead girls, Alice Marsh and Emma Shrivell. The letter purported to warn them against a Dr. Harper who, if they didn't watch out, would serve them as he had Matilda Clover and Lou Harvey. What most intrigued the sergeant about the letter was the name Lou Harvey. There was nothing in the file to the effect that a girl with that name had been poisoned.

The result of Cream's visit was that detectives were ordered to follow him while others went looking for Lou Harvey on the theory that she must have met the murderer but hadn't taken the lethal pill and, unknown to the killer, had survived.

Cream had a drinking friend named John Haynes, and it was Haynes who pointed out the fact to Cream as they left the boarding house one day that somebody, who looked like a policeman, was following him. Cream didn't show concern. He replied,

"I know about all that. It's a medical student named Harper they're watching for – he poisoned all those whores."

"If you know anything about it," Haynes warned, "you should go to the police and tell them."

"I think there's more money to be made by telling Dr. Harper, the boy's father, what I know."

Later, they were riding on a bus when they heard a newsboy shouting, "Arrest in the Stamford Street case! Read all about it." Haynes said that Cream became violently excited about this, and wanted to jump off the bus there and then.

When they left the bus at Charing Cross, Cream skidded across the road like a demented animal and bought the entire stock of a newsboy's papers. Cream's relief on discovering the story referred to another crime in the notorious Stamford Street area was reminiscent of a gout-sufferer coming out of pain.

On May 26, Cream had a caller at his lodgings. It was Detective-Inspector Tunbridge of the CID. He was the epitome of politeness. He told Cream he had been put in charge of the Stamford Street murders, was sorry to trouble him, but might he have any ideas or any knowledge of the disturbing mystery? Cream, who warmed to an audience – even if it might prove a dangerous and hostile one – became talkative. He produced a bottle of strychnine tablets. "I think, inspector, you will find that your quarry is a man of medicine – for only doctors can buy pills like these."

Cream used the occasion to complain that policemen were following him about. "There's probably one in the street opposite waiting for me to go for a walk right now."

"Oh." Tunbridge expressed horror and promised to look into the matter and raise the issue on Cream's behalf.

"You had better see Young Harper," Cream said with biting sarcasm, "I'm sure he can tell you more than I can."

Tunbridge saw Harper junior. More important, however, was the fact that he took the trouble to take the train to Barnstable and see Dr. Harper senior. When the doctor showed Tunbridge the threatening letter he had received, Tunbridge said, "I think you have there, sir, the very thing I want. If I'm not mistaken, that's Dr. Cream's handwriting and he's our suspect."

Tunbridge had not been appointed to the case the day before; he had been working on it for some weeks. The problem was that the girls who could identify Cream were mostly illiterate young prostitutes, and it was doubtful if anything they said would convince a jury. Constable Crumley who had seen Emma Shrivell let Cream out of the Stamford Street house had recognised him coming from a music hall. But again, as with the girls, Crumley had only seen Cream late at night; gaslight was poor, so would a jury accept this testimony? Tunbridge was looking for letters – especially the really damaging ones Cream had written to the girls making appointments. But the cunning Cream had foreseen this and had always had the girls return them before delivering the *coup de grace*.

But the letter purporting to come from Murray, while not evidence of murder, was sufficient to charge Cream with something else.

Material witnesses were not only few, but usually they were dead. It was true that Cream had already shown the police he had previous knowledge that strychnine had killed Matilda Clover – and this a month before she was exhumed and found to have died from the poison. But, puzzling to us now, the police thought the evidence was insufficient to secure a conviction. This might very well have been a reflection of the class-structure climate of the times. Cream was a gentleman, even if he was an eccentric and slightly barmy one. The victims weren't really important people. They weren't even members of the deserving poor class, but outcasts, misfits, rejects, a nuisance, and many thought a disgrace to the city. Whatever the police might have thought, there was the jury to consider, twelve every-day men and women of a social order somewhat below Dr. Cream's.

But Tunbridge had irrefutable evidence with the letter received by Dr. Harper – evidence not of murder, but evidence to warrant a charge of attempted blackmail, extortion and demanding money with menaces. This would hold Cream behind bars while the more important investigation was pursued.

Cream was arrested on June 3. "You've got the wrong man," he screamed at Tunbridge. Then, his manner changing abruptly, he lifted his arms in resignation as if facing a firing squad and said, "Fire away."

There was an inquest on Matilda and the jury found Cream guilty of her wilful murder and, in October, Cream stood in the Old Bailey, appearing for the third time on trial for his life. He was confident that he would escape the gallows as he had done before because, apart from the letters, the evidence against him didn't prove to be all that significant. Also there were those in court who thought he would escape, particularly as his wealth had provided him with the best defence lawyers. He was cool to the point of insolence in court and, for once, had nothing to say about the crimes. On the last day of the trial, his counsel gave such an impressive performance in his final speech that Cream accepted the good wishes of his guards and danced and sang with glee in his cell that night.

But the jury found him guilty and after he had been sentened to death, he muttered, "They shall never hang me." He was wrong again – they did. It happened less than a month after his trial.

On his last day, he could not sleep but paced his cell restlessly throughout the night. It was thought that he would make a last minute confession, but he denied committing the murders, and was hanged leaving the mystery behind him of what had really been his motive for his cruel and pointless crimes.

DR. ROBERT BUCHANAN

By the very commission of the crime, murderers are revealing a collection of character defects – ultra-egotism, callousness and immorality being among them – but I think it would be correct to say that a lack of courage isn't usually among their failings. When a murderer does lack nerves of steel, however, you get the macabre comedy Dr. Robert Buchanan committed in New York in 1892.

There's probably been no jittier killer than Dr. Buchanan and the quaking he did in public after committing the crime – which had been the perfect murder and went undetected – soon attracted interest from the police. It reached the height of absurdity when he employed a private detective to guard his wife's grave, fearing that the authorities would exhume her and discover the skilful blending of poisons in her stomach.

Courage wasn't a fact he considered when planning the killing; either he lacked confidence in his ability to plan and kill or his conscience, another unknown factor before the crime, reared to smash him afterwards. Whatever the motivation, the doctor became so convinced that people were watching him, whispering about him, telling others about him, that he became a nervous wreck, a man haunted. Hiring a private detective to guard the grave in a public cemetery was followed by the appointment of a lawyer to defend him before anybody suspected murder. With such odd behaviour, even to the point of stopping people on the street and asking them if they had heard rumours about a doctor murdering his wife, there could only be one conclusion – suspicion, investigation, exhumation, post mortem, and arrest.

Dr. Buchanan, attractive, once well-dressed and fastidious, shambled nervously off to jail with one satisfaction in his mind. He had been right all the time. People had been plotting against him. He didn't discover until his trial that it was his own erratic behaviour which had brought him down. There had been gossip, of course, and one of the first to bear malice was a shifty-eyed brothel-bouncer named Smith. He called at the shabby offices of Louis Schultze, the New York Coroner one afternoon in May 1892.

He said he had come to tell about a murder which nobody seemed to know about since the victim had been buried without any fuss and because her demise had been accredited to normal causes. Mr. Schultze wasn't impressed. He had heard such stories before and usually a cursory investigation was sufficient to show the informant was inspired by malice, revenge, hope of financial reward or fame – or because he was crazy.

But Smith said his piece. Until eighteen months before, he said, he had been employed as a bouncer in a brothel. It was a modest ten-girl house in Newark, New Jersey, and the madame's name had been Annie Sutherland. Smith had been in love with Annie. She was, he said, "Fat and fifty, not much to look at, but she had a heart of gold." And then a cruel thing happened. Annie had suddenly upped and married one of the house's regular patrons, closed the business – putting Smith out of work – and gone to live in Greenwich Village. Annie's husband was the fastidious Dr. Buchanan who was twenty years her junior and a man with whom she had nothing in common.

Schultze remained unimpressed believing that when sex reared its head the most unlikely events can occur. But Smith persisted. Even Annie's friends had remarked on Annie's gutter coarseness and lack of sophistication; the doctor, educated, cultured, and meticulous was clearly of a much higher class.

With the curious puritanism of the brothel-bouncer Smith complained that Buchanan had worked his way through each of the girls in the brothel before developing his love for "Ma Annie." The theory among the other girls, as the doctor wooed Annie with gifts of chocolates and flowers and invitations to dinner, was that he was after her money.

So after the wedding and the sale of the Newark house, Smith decided to investigate Buchanan. The doctor lived on West 11th Street, and Smith had uncovered a great deal of local gossip. He discovered for instance that Buchanan's first wife – who he had met and married in Nova Scotia – had recently divorced him because of his many infidelities. She had returned to Halifax with all the money and the doctor's practice, because of his behaviour with his women patients, had suffered badly.

Annie Sutherland, world-worn and shrewd, had gone to pieces when the doctor began wooing her, seeing in him the opportunity to acquire the polish and position that life had denied her. "Annie wouldn't hear a thing said against the doc," said Smith.

"But none of his patients were safe. The other wives in the neighbourhood told his first wife, but the final break came when

119

she came down to the surgery one night from their apartment above, and found the doc at it on the carpet."

After her marriage to Buchanan, Annie kept in touch with a few of the girls. And what shocked Smith was that Buchanan also kept in surreptitious touch with one of them. Soon Smith was hearing tales of marital friction; Annie, it was said, was maintaining angrily that she wouldn't give Buchanan another nickel until he treated her like a lady, a wife, and with the respect her position deserved.

Defending Buchanan, the girl whom the doctor was secretly seeing, told Smith and the other girls just what he had to put up with. She quoted what he had told her: "You have no idea what an ordeal my honeymoon with Annie was like," he was quoted as saying. "God, but Annie's coarse. She swears like a trooper and she tells blue stories in genteel company,"

Smith told the Coroner that Annie *was* coarse and common and swore like an old sweat, "But is that a crime? Is that an excuse to murder her?"

Coroner Schultze had made the right noises. It added up, he thought, to an interesting story – juicy was the word. He agreed that the doctor's interest in Annie had obviously been her money, but he didn't see that Smith's story pointed to murder.

Either Coroner Schultze introduced Smith to a reporter named Ike White or the bouncer, seeing that he wouldn't get any satisfaction from the coroner, went *looking* for the reporter. Ike White was one of the new breed of journalists who catered for the reading needs of the newly-literate masses. He worked for Joseph Pulitzer, the blind publisher of the New York *World*, who was pioneering the yellow press school of reporting, and was soon to have an even more sensational rival with William Randolph Hearst's *Journal*. The stable diet of the yellow press was an unending supply of scandal and exposé, from graft in government to vice in squalid places. If at times the exposé wasn't always justifiable at least the reporter's motives were claimed to be pure and a great deal of injustice was aired in the open.

White already had a reputation. He had made himself famous in a recent poisoning case which had led to a New York medical student named Carlyle Harris being sentenced to death for the murder of his wife. Coroner Schultze had officiated at the original inquest and had ruled accidental death through an overdose of morphine. It had looked as if Harris would get away with it, but White, carrying out an exhaustive investigation, had got to the truth and had told all in a page-one scoop which had embarrassed the coroner and the police. When White heard what Smith had to say about Whorehouse Annie and the dapper doctor his pen hand began to itch as he wondered if lightning could strike a second time in the same place.

White visited Greenwich Village and discovered that Buchanan, who was a heavy drinker, had drunk regularly at Michael Macomber's bar on 10th Street. Not revealing his identity he began to frequent Macomber's, and soon discovered that Buchanan was well-known there. It was an unprepossessing bar and Macomber was proud of the fact that such a well-dressed and prominent man such as Dr. Buchanan used his establishment and that he was his close friend.

White discovered that after Annie's death, the doctor had returned to Halifax, Nova Scotia, in an attempt to get over the tragedy, but Macomber thought he would shortly be back. White contacted a reporter in Halifax and received some startling news. As soon as he arrived in Halifax, Buchanan had gone calling on his divorced wife and in a trice had remarried her. The reporter also said that Buchanan was putting it about in Halifax that he had to return to New York because he had large financial holdings there.

During his evenings in the bar White heard much corrobative gossip from the talkative Macomber and the other drinkers. Macomber said he had liked Annie but the doctor was much too good for her. Everybody it seemed thought the same.

"Annie sure was coarse, mister," Macomber said. "And they don't come any louder and coarser. She could stand at the other end of the bar on a busy night and you'd hear her cursing through all the noise right at the other end." Macomber added that the poor doctor used to wilt in embarrassment under the flood of language.

With such an ill match, Macomber claimed, friction was soon showing itself and the couple were quarrelling in public. The pattern was invariably the same. Buchanan complained about Annie's vulgarity, and Annie complained that her husband didn't treat her like a lady. Buchanan would retort that he couldn't treat her like a lady if she didn't act like one.

Eventually, the story went, the doctor stopped bringing Annie to the bar. He would drop in alone and soon Macomber noticed that he had the habit of taking his meals in the tavern. When Macomber had asked him why he didn't eat at home since he now had a wife, Dr. Buchanan had claimed – and seemed to be serious about it – that Annie was trying to poison him. Later, he told the proprietor that Annie was a morphine addict and would kill herself if she didn't break the habit. When he heard the magic word *morphine*, the effect on reporter White was electric. Morphine had been used in the recent murder case he had exposed in which the medical student had tried to create the impression that the girl he had secretly married had killed herself accidentally. Since the trial had been well-publicised White began to wonder if Buchanan had got the idea from the newspapers.

White kept the drinks and the questions flowing and then Macomber, in all innocence, revealed further gossip of a damaging nature. The heart-broken Dr. Buchanan had been in such a hurry to get poor Annie buried that he had made the arrangements over night in the bar and invited some casual drinking cronies to the funeral. With that heavy mawkishness which can hang over a bar like a cloud of tobacco smoke at midnight, the bar-proppers rallied around the broken-hearted doctor and offered their services as pallbearers. Annie was hastened off to Greenwood Cemetery, Brooklyn, on April 26, 1892, with no friend, relative or even an ex-Newark whorehouse employee to accompany her, but carried there by a host of unsalubrious bar-room strangers who had been forcibly sobered-up for the occasion. Well might White have wondered which of the two had been vulgar beneath the surface – Annie or Buchanan.

It was these same whisky-sinkers who gave the reporter further startling information when he joined them in their drinking marathons. White casually mentioned the Harris poison case in conversation to see if it brought a reaction, and it paid off in a good way. Harris had been a dope, Macomber said with a chuckle for with the right blending of poisons he could have got away with it. White asked him what he meant since he had no medical knowledge, and as White guessed he would, Macomber fell to quoting Dr. Buchanan.

Dr. Buchanan had been in the bar almost every day while the trial dragged on and had explained the medical aspects of it to his friends. On the day Harris had been found guilty, Buchanan had been most contemptuous about the medical student, and had said, "It's easy to get away with murder by using morphine because, in chemistry, every acid has its base, and every agent its reagent." Buchanan hadn't enlarged on this remark because it was too abstruse to explain to knuckleheads.

White also checked Annie's will at the probate court and discovered that all her wealth, amounting to some eighteen thousand dollars, had been left to the doctor. He next collected a copy of the death certificate and found her death had been attributed to a stroke. White then called on a doctor named McIntire, who had attended to Annie in her final illness and had signed the certificate. On reflection, McIntire told him, some of the symptoms Annie had shown in her illness were consistent with morphine poisoning; but – and it was a big but – one crucial symptom which showed up only in morphine poisoning was missing. This was a narrowing of the pupils of the eyes to mere pinpricks. Since Annie's pupils had been normal, McIntire said, death had to be due to something else, and all the symptoms pointed to cerebral haemorrhage. The doctor refused to accept that Annie had been poisoned with morphine even after hearing all what White had to say about Buchanan. He maintained that the pupils would not have remained normal had Annie died from the drug.

White checked this with other doctors and got the same answer. He was forced to switch to other assignments but, still believing that he was right, he returned to Macomber's bar when he could spare the time. One night he arrived there to find a celebration in progress. It was occasioned by the return of Dr. Buchanan, who sat in the seat of honour. White joined the party and was introduced.

Reporter White observed several things during the drinking session. He noticed that the doctor drank more than anybody else in the company of hard drinkers. He noticed, too, that at times Buchanan had some big problem on his mind. His hands would begin to quiver and he would look repeatedly at the door. White knew he was looking at a man who was haunted by fright.

The first Mrs. Buchanan – now the third, although she didn't know it – had also noticed peculiarities in her husband's behaviour. These developed as soon as they arrived in New York. It was as if Buchanan had an allergy to the place. He looked both ill and worried. Her story, as she would later tell it, was that Buchanan had called to see her as soon as he arrived in Halifax. He had said nothing about his second marriage – just that he was lonely, missing her, demanded her forgiveness and begged her to marry him again. She agreed but nobody was more surprised than she when, after the service, he said they must pack and return to New York. She thought he hated New York, but he now claimed he had important business arrangements in the city and if he wasn't there, people would conspire to rob him.

Since he wished to keep his second marriage secret, it is surprising he went back to the old home on 11th street – where both his first wife and, later, Annie had lived with him and where both had gossiped with the neighbours. As soon as they arrived in New York, Dr. Buchanan's behaviour became more irrational. He begged her not to go out of the house unless he was with her, and he insisted that she did not talk to the neighbours unless he was present. If Mrs. Buchanan thought about this, she possibly presumed that her husband had carried on wildly in her absence and didn't want the gossipers telling her about the girls who had stayed there.

But it was while he was talking to Buchanan in the bar, White later recalled, that it dawned on him how Buchanan had poisoned Annie with morphine and had escaped detection. *Every acid has a base, every agent its reagent.* He was looking directly at the doctor and the doctor had bad eyesight which meant he wore glasses. The lenses of his spectacles were so thickly magnified that the pupils of his eyes looked enlarged. While he talked, White reflected on this. He remembered something from his childhood. A school friend had gone for an eye test and to facilitate this the optician had placed atrophine drops in his eyes which had made his pupils enlarge for a time. The big question was: had Buchanan dosed his wife's eyes with atrophine while he was poisoning her so that McIntire wouldn't see the pupils contracted to pinpricks which would have immediately warned him that she was being poisoned with morphine.

The more he thought about this, the more White was convinced he was on the right track. He went back to call on a nurse who had attended Annie in her final illness. He had learned nothing from her in their last talk, but now he knew what he was after. Yes, the nurse finally said, Dr. Buchanan had on several occasions placed something in his wife's eyes. She said he had done it several times a day. White returned to the coroner, Louis Schultze, who agreed that White had gathered a great weight of circumstantial evidence. A conference was called to look into the matter and to see if there was justification in calling for an exhumation and a post mortem.

But now Michael Macomber and the drinking boys were commenting on Buchanan's peculiar behaviour. Every day brought a fresh crop of stories. Dr. Buchanan had stopped a stranger in the street and asked him if he had heard any gossip to the effect that a doctor in the neighbourhood had poisoned his wife. He was convinced now that people were saying he had murdered Annie and he asked his drinking pals if they could really believe that he would do a thing like that. Macomber became worried. He told the doctor to take a firm hold of himself.The cronies were beginning to look at Buchanan in an odd way, for they were beginning to realise the truth of the old saying *There's no smoke without fire.*

Buchanan finally went to pieces. He carried out three actions which were damning. He hired a private detective named Hood to go out to the cemetery and guard Annie's grave. If anybody tried to dig up the coffin, the man must hurry to the doctor and let him know. He changed his address, went into hiding – and only told

Hood where he would be – and never mentioned to his wife where he was going. Buchanan also called on a lawyer and paid him a hundred dollars to defend him should he get into trouble. The lawyer asked him if he had done anything, and Buchanan said, "I might be accused of poisoning my second wife." The lawyer asked him if he had, and Buchanan said, "Of course not, but you know how people like to talk."

The authorities found Hood, the private detective, when they went to the cemetery to exhume Annie. He was hovering about near her grave. Hood said, "I don't know why he wants me to watch it. All I've got to do is tell him if anybody tries to open it. Sure, it's a crazy assignment, but, goddamnit, I needed the money." Hood told the police where Buchanan was living, and detectives were placed near the house to follow him until he was arrested. The autopsy was something of an anticlimax. It confirmed a fatal amount of morphine in Annie's body and though atrophine was no longer present in the eyes, there was nothing to indicate that it hadn't been used.

Dr. Buchanan was arrested on June 7. His apprehension left him as soon as he was in jail and he became his old, confident and bumptious self. "Annie was trying to poison me with morphine," he said, "and I suggest she made a mistake, got the plates mixed, and took the lethal dose herself."

As has happened in so many murder poison trials, there was a terrific battle in court with qualified medical men taking up a stance on either side. For every doctor who attempted to show that Buchanan was guilty, the defence produced one to try and show that he was not. And for a long time it looked as if the dapper doctor would get away with it.

One of the doctor's defence lawyers was William J. O'Sullivan, who was unknown until he defended Buchanan. As a result of the case he became famous overnight. Prior to taking up law, he had been a physician, and he knew enough about poisons and doctors to put up an argument in favour of Buchanan. In the six months before the trial came round, O'Sullivan researched and gained much more knowledge about toxicology. He was beginning to realise why juries in Europe had been reluctant to convict for murder on scientific evidence alone. Perhaps judges and juries were fussy, but they liked to have concrete evidence before assuming guilt. They preferred to have competent witnesses step forward and say that they had seen the accused purchase the poison or had witnessed him or her administer it.

O'Sullivan got medical backing for his researches and tests were carried out. After the prosecution's medical experts had had their say, all stipulating that morphine in fatal quantities had been found in Annie, O'Sullivan brought in his tamed scientists. Put simply, O'Sullivan's case was that a decomposing body produces its own poison. These are known as cadaveric alkaloids. Having reminded everybody on that, he said that these reacted the same way in tests as did morphine. What the autopsy said was that the morphine in Annie's body was really a poison produced by decay. O'Sullivan's experts had carried out tests to support his argument with dead animals, and he laid on a medical test in court – with white-frocked scientists and laboratory paraphernalia – to demonstrate his argument was valid. He caused a sensation. It made front page in the newspapers across the world. Down in the Macomber bar on 10th street, the boys made whoopee and prepared to welcome the doctor's return.

But in their jubilation, Buchanan's defence made a mistake, which cost the doctor his life. To strengthen their case for an acquittal, they decided that Buchanan should go into the witness box. If he didn't go in, they argued, the jury might think he was frightened to stand up to cross examination and it might damage his chances. So into the box, with all his cockiness, went Dr. Buchanan. A few hard questions touched him where it hurt most, on his conscience, and in the merciless interrogation from the prosecution Buchanan told so many lies that he almost tied his tongue in knots, and ended up by contradicting everything he had said before. O'Sullivan's brilliant scientific defence was soon washed away in a flood of lies and although it took them twenty-eight hours to dc so, the jury found Buchanan guilty and he was sentenced to death. It was only down at a shabby little bar on 10th street that you could find a hard-core of people who maintained Doc Buchanan had been framed.

CARLYLE HARRIS

If a tempestuous medical student named Carlyle Harris hadn't fallen in love he wouldn't have committed murder, nor would Dr. Buchanan have got the idea not only to imitate him but to try and improve upon his method. Young, handsome and dashing, Carl Harris was in his third year at the New York College of Surgeons and Physicians, when he came face to face with a problem that destroyed his appetite and kept him awake at night. He was in love with a pretty teenager named Helen Potts but, in keeping with the moral climate of the time, Helen wouldn't yield the flower-token of love until he'd slipped that little band of gold on her dainty finger.

What could Harris do? There were several good solid family reasons why he couldn't, or shouldn't, marry the girl, and they came under the general headings of class distinctions and restrictive customs. Miss Potts, who lived on Ocean Grove, definitely came from the sticks, while Carl was the grandson of snooty Benjamin McCready, a prominent New York professor of medicine. His mother was straight-laced and very aware of her station in life. She was a frequent lecturer for one of the temperance societies, but of the better sort, of course. Perhaps closer investigation would have shown that the Harris family weren't really blue-blooded at all, and perhaps this was the core of the problem, for the watery blue are often snootier than the genuinely blue. Neither his grandfather nor his mother would take to unsophisticated Helen, that was one thing that the jittery Carl was sure of. Even if they could develop a warmth for the girl he loved, Mother Potts was something else again. It appeared she had to be seen to be believed. Moreover he relied on his family, particularly his grandfather for his fees. How could he saddle the man with an extra mouth to feed without getting his approval first?

Carl had met Helen on a holiday in New Jersey a year before he married her. They met in dusty libraries, gloomy museums and remote cafes, during this year of frustration.

"Please, Helen."

"No, darling. You must be strong and wait. If we do, we'll never go to Heaven. Ma says I shouldn't. Your family will say the same."

Hot blood is a spur to quick thought and in the cold winter of 1890, when Carl was really sickened by hand-clasps and stolen kisses in draughty museums, he got what he thought was a bright idea. He would marry Helen and insist for the time being that they keep the marriage a secret. He produced valid reasons for Helen as to why they should keep the truth from his family. For example he wasn't yet working so couldn't support her, and since he had no money it would be an imposition for him to expect his family to do so. Much better surely, he argued, to wait until he had his own independence when, with his own income flowing in, he would have the right to do what he liked. That would be the time to introduce Helen to his family. We don't know what the boy had at the back of his mind during this period. Carl's hot blood blinded him to potential dangers. He wanted Helen now and would let the future take care of itself.

Carl was a smooth talker. He would have played up the romantic aspects of a secret marriage. "It's just like an elopement, darling." Helen was satisfied. Apparently she didn't need much convincing and why should she, for it was a step in the right direction even if it wasn't a complete step. But Carl had to finish his education before he got married, so it seemed both sensible and right to her to keep their union a secret. Besides it was so excitingly romantic and wouldn't it be fun to share such a big secret?

One cold wintery day Helen wrapped herself up warmly and told her mother that Carl was taking her on a sight-seeing tour of the New York stock exchange. Mrs. Potts knew Carl. Helen brought him round for tea after which, at a decent hour, poor Carl had to trudge home through the cold and think of Helen all snugged up alone in her bed. Mrs. Potts liked Carl and thought he would be a fine husband – better than she could hope for – for her daughter. But she was troubled by their sharply contrasting backgrounds and must have guessed that the Harris family would be against the marriage. The fact that Carl had never taken Helen to see his mother or grandfather seemed confirmation of this, and she hoped that Helen, sweet and innocent, wasn't going to end up being badly hurt.

The couple didn't go to the stock exchange. Instead they slipped into dim, dark and dusty City Hall where an alderman, with a bad cold and dandruff, hustled them through a marriage ceremony. To keep the reporters from sniffing around, Harris went down in the books as common Charles Harris and his wife as

Helen Neilson Potts. Because Helen was a little disappointed by the shabbiness of it all, Carl whispered, "Don't worry, darling. We'll do it again, in church, and with more style – eventually." Then he hustled her off to the sticky warmth of a hotel.

Because of certain domestic arrangements the couple had to make, Mrs Potts had to be informed. She was both surprised and delighted and, at first, she saw the need for secrecy. She agreed that Carl needed to be independent before the announcement was made, and admired the pride he showed in not expecting his family to set him and Helen up in their first home.

The marriage took place on February 8, 1890, and exactly a year later – less a week – it would be alleged that the embryo doctor had murdered his young wife, alleged because not everybody would believe that it actually was murder. Meanwhile the expectable unexpected soon happened, and Helen found that she was pregnant.

Helen anxiously told Carl that now they must reveal the truth and announce they were married, but Carl said he had a better way. Persuasively he convinced her that it was too soon for them to have a baby, and that he was determined not to go to his family for help. It is hard to believe that the family were really as bad as Harris claimed them to be, and it is probable that much of their coldness was imagination or just stubborn independence and pride on his part. He suggested that he carry out an abortion, which would be safe as he was almost a doctor. Helen allowed him to do it. He botched it and Helen, now seriously ill, was packed off by Mrs. Potts to a relative in the country, who was a doctor. There during the summer she had a premature child who was dead at birth. Then still ill and suffering from migraine headaches, she returned to New York and her husband.

Mrs. Potts thought the time had come for the secret to emerge. She wanted Helen to have a church marriage, but Harris begged smoothly for a few months delay, after which time he would have graduated. Meantime, he had another brilliant idea. While they waited, Helen should go to a finishing school for gentle ladies and this would make her more presentable to his family. Harris said he knew the very place: Miss Lydia Day's school, the Comstock, at 32 West Fortieth Street. She could be a boarder there and he could introduce her to his family while on visits away from the school. Since they knew the school's reputation they would be impressed by any girl Harris brought home from there. After a few meetings, said Carl, he could either tell his family the truth or just have a second marriage, in church, without having to mention the first.

Mrs. Potts had grave doubts, and she raised a couple of them.

Carl was smooth and she told him sarcastically, "Any more bright ideas?" She wondered what he was playing at. The Potts might be nobodies but they were still respectable God-fearing nobodies. She wanted Helen married in church and all the world, should the world be interested, to know about it. But cunningly Carl convinced her. If his motives had earlier been genuine it was now, according to his later detractors, that they ceased to be so. Now, if not before, he tired of the situation and wanted to be rid of Helen, and not have his family know anything about her. Helen was pale and ill, a sharp contrast in every way to the bright, carefree girls he had met in his own social circle while she had been in the country. Carl now prescribed pills for Helen's recurring headaches. He wrote a prescription for six capsules. Each contained 4–1/6th grains of quinine and 1/6th grains of morphine. This, a standard medicine in those lax times, was made up by McIntyre & Sons of Sixth Avenue.

It would be alleged at his trial for murder that he emptied one of these tablets and refilled it with pure morphine, and that he gave it, with three of the other pills, to Helen. At the same time, it was said that he kept two back so that he could produce them after her death for analysis in order to show that they were harmless. Carl instructed Helen to take one pill before going to bed when ever she felt particularly bad.

Helen went off to the school for gentle ladies with this medical version of Russian roulette. Three times she was lucky. Three times she dipped her fingers into her little pillbox and took out a harmless capsule. Then she came home for a weekend's leave. Packing her case before returning to the school, she found the last pill.

"I don't think I'll take this, ma. They're not doing me any good." She was about to throw it away when her mother interrupted her. Everybody can look back on a statement which they wished they had never made. Marie Antoinette probably regretted saying that if the people didn't have bread they should eat cake, and Neville Chamberlain, back from Munich and Hitler, that he had brought a piece of paper which meant that there would be peace in our time.

Thus poor Mrs Potts was to regret her line to Helen. "Oh, do take it with you, Helen. You may need it. And Carl's the doctor and knows best."

The girls were going to a symphony concert but, feeling low, Helen said she would go to bed early instead. She was sleeping when her roommates returned and they awoke her. "Oh, I had a fantastic dream," she told them. The morphine was already working on her. "I wished it could have gone on forever. I've never had anything like it."

"Was Carl in it?" they asked playfully.

The girls knew Carl, although they didn't know about the marriage. Carl visited the school when he came to collect Helen for the evening.

"Oh, yes, Carl was there."

Later, after the lights were out, one of them heard Helen moaning. The girls put on the lights and went to see what was wrong. Helen said she couldn't breath and kept feeling as if she was choking. One of her roommates stroked her hair and face and then Helen said she couldn't feel the girl's fingers. Later still she said she thought she was going to die and asked, "Do you think that the medicine Carl gave me could do me harm?"

By now she was finding it so hard to breath that the girls went for the headmistress. This was at midnight. Mrs Day, finding Helen unconscious, sent for a physician, Dr. E. P. Fowler, who lived a few doors away. He found Helen in a coma, her flesh blue tinted, her skin cold to the touch. He immediately noticed that the pupils of her eyes had narrowed to the size of pinheads, an indication of morphine poisoning. Eventually he called in two other doctors and they fought throughout the night and late into the next day to save the girl.

The doctors used atropine, caffeine and all the restoratives they could think of. They also used artificial respiration. When he could, Dr Fowler carried out a search of Helen's belongings, puzzled by the poisoning. He found the empty pillbox. It gave the name of the drug store and added, underneath, "for C. W. H." He called to Miss Day – "Who's C. W. H.?"

"I think the initials must stand for Mr Carlyle Harris. He's Helen's friend. He's also a medical student."

Dr Fowler promptly sent for Harris, and it was dawn before he arrived. He told Dr Fowler that the pills had consisted of one sixth morphine and the rest quinine. Then Harris said something which the doctor thought rather odd at the time, for it indicated a selfishness and callousness ill-fitted for the fact that the girl, whom he supposedly loved was unconscious and probably dying on the nearby bed. "Doctor, do you think I could be held responsible?"

Fowler told him bitterly, "I think, young man, that you should hurry round to McIntyre's and check whether a mistake was made."

Harris appeared eager to be gone to carry out this mission. However, a telling point against him at his trial, was that he didn't go to the druggist. Was he frightened because he knew that there had been no mistake? He used up time by aimlessly walking the streets and then returned and told the doctors that there had been no error.

Helen would remain alive, but in a coma, for another four hours while the doctors fought fruitlessly to save her. Harris's contribution was that they should perform a tracheotomy – cut the windpipe and insert a breathing tube – but Dr Fowler said this would kill Helen instantly. At noon he announced that she was dead, and the three doctors looked pointedly at a crestfallen Harris as they left the room.

Harris didn't go to the funeral in New Jersey because, as he told Mrs. Potts, "I know I will only break down and make a spectacle of myself."

The secret marriage was kept from the coroner, Louis Schultze (who would also figure in the Buchanan case); and while he was aware that morphine had caused the death, he couldn't see any motive for foul play. Who would want to kill a pretty young girl? It was illogical. Since he didn't call for a post mortem nobody knew how much morphine was in Helen's body. He found that death had been caused by an unfortunate accident. Either, he declared, the pharmacy had made a mistake by putting too much morphine in one of the capsules or Helen had disobeyed Harris's instructions and had taken more than one capsule at a time. In either case, Helen's heart hadn't been able to fight against the increased dosage. The coroner saw no reason to spend public money on an autopsy under these circumstances.

The matter, judged an accidental death, was closed. Harris left the court after having his knuckles gently rapped for prescribing drugs before his licence to practice came through.

But there had been talk, whispers, and Ike White, a reporter on the *World*, heard them. The muck-raking *World* was always on the look out for a juicy scandal, and though tiresome, a scandal sheet occasionally justifies its existance by coming up with gold from the mud. White discovered that Harris was a member of the nororious *Neptune Club* – its secretary no less. One of the foundations of the club, inexcusable in those times, was that it believed in a permissive society and there was talk of orgies on the premises. A juicy yarn about the goings-on of the rich and fashionable, therefore, seemed to have been White's initial spur to investigate the case further. He met Mrs Potts who let out the fact of the secret marriage for the first time. White already thought that the coroner should have had an autopsy and now he realised that there had indeed been a motive for murder. Harris had a wife he might very well have tired of but couldn't be rid of legally without a scandal.

To keep up a façade of respectability was probably the motive for scores of Victorian murders that we have never heard about. This seems to have been the reason in Harris's case and was certainly so in County Cork, where Dr Cross had murdered his wife just three years before.

What added punch to White's investigation, was the fact that Harris's mother at her religious and temperance meetings, frequently held up her son as a shining example of the paragon of virtue that can be found in a good religious and abstemious home. The truth, however, White believed was to be found in the *Neptune Club*, where seductions were achieved by plying girls, it was said, with gingerpop heavily laced with whisky. And now he had discovered all about the secret marriage which was so closely followed by that fatal overdose from a drug provided by Helen's secret husband. White's story made page-one in the *World*, and the outcry that followed was so intense that the authorities had to order an autopsy.

A prominent toxicologist, Dr Rudolph Witthaus, found enough morphine in Helen's body to kill her but, oddly, no quinine. The next logical step was to have Harris arrested. The case against him was largely circumstantial, more plausible argument than incriminating fact. The prosecution, at his trial, claimed he ordered the capsules from a leading pharmacy and then kept back two so that if, as happened, Helen took the fatal one last, he could show by the name of the pharmacy and by tests conducted on the remaining pills that the drugs had indeed been harmless.

But the scheme, said the prosecution, worked both ways, and that it had in fact, boomeranged against Harris. Since the two drugs produced by Harris were harmless, the jury should therefore presume that the other four, unless tampered with, were also harmless. The phamarcist would hardly have put more morphine in one pill than in the others, and the two samples they had investigated had contained finely measured amounts. If this fact could not be accepted as conclusive proof, then nor could Harris's reason for only giving Helen four of the drugs. According to him he held back two pills because he didn't want her to have too many at one time.

Picking up this point, his defence lawyers raised the possibility that Helen had committed suicide, either by saving up all the drugs and taking them at once, or by getting morphine from elsewhere. But Miss Day and her schoolfriends had already testified to her happy disposition. Before going to bed that fatal night, Helen had cheerfully read John Brown's *Talks About Dogs* to Miss Day. Nor did suicide fit with the testimony of the girls who had heard Helen's last words before she slipped into the coma.

The public were divided into two camps as to whether Harris had murdered Helen or not. Daily reports were studied avidly as the court hearing got more and more bogged down by the contradictory arguments from medical experts for both the prosecution and for the defence. As usual in these acrimonious debates, the jury suffered and, as often happens, refused in the end to accept medical evidence from either side.

Harris's chief defence lawyer, William Travers Jerome, (who was to collapse from strain during the protracted trial) tried to discredit Dr Witthaus's testimony. He prepared for the attack by researching into cadaveric alkaloids – poisons produced by the body after death – and then tried to establish the fact that a great many poisons existed which nobody yet knew about. Dr. Witthaus firmly maintained that he had applied every known test in order to establish that morphine was the cause of death, even to the point of carrying out research on frogs.

Jerome then attempted to show that the morphine content of the last capsule, a sixth of a grain, could have been sufficient in itself to kill Helen. The weakness in this argument was that Helen had earlier taken three similar drugs and survived. Jerome soon changed his tactics by next suggesting that Helen had an unknown kidney complaint which could have caused her death. The prosecution then called on medical opinion to debate this point and to adjudge that if Helen had indeed had a kidney complaint whether it could have killed her. The Harris family were putting up a bundle for his defence and the lawyers were going to do their best to earn it. In their opinion the judge wasn't interfering enough to see that the hearing remained on the right and probable course. The only thing that Jerome hadn't so far suggested was that the man in the moon might have dropped down and popped a pill into the sleeping girl's mouth.

Two druggists from McIntyre's demonstrated how the pills were prepared and the safety devices and the double checking system which was used, and which made it impossible for accidents to occur. Although the evidence against him was largely circumstantial, the jury took only an hour to find Harris guilty. He was sentenced to death. The Court of Appeals and the Governor of New York reexamined the case and concurred with the findings. It is doubtful if the evidence today would be considered conclusive enough in either an English or an American court to bring such a verdict, especially as the death penalty was called for. In England Harris might very well have got away with the benefit of the doubt. In the States also, especially with the more tricky lawyers available today, and with the funds of a wealthy family behind him Harris might well be set free.

The puritanism, which has often marred justice in these two countries, undoubtedly helped convict Harris in the minds of the jury, if not of the judges. It seemed that they decided that a man who would ply girls with strong drink and participate in orgies, was also the type who would commit murder.

The prosecution had also introduced a witness, a friend of Harris, who alleged that Harris had told him that he would kill both Helen and himself rather than have his family find out about his marriage. Harris's fear of his grandfather seemed to be genuine, even if it was unnecessary. It was a time of parental tyranny.

Harris was beholden to his grandfather both for his college fees and for pocket money, and young men did not marry until they could support a wife and family. Any connection with a girl which went beyond hand touching and cheek kissing was definitely illicit. Moreover, since marriage was something the respectable did only once in a life-time, (and a doctor must be beyond reproach), Harris was stuck with Helen – unless she died. These were the thoughts which convinced the jury.

Evidence against Harris also said that he had had an hectic affair with a girl whom he had tried to persuade to marry a wealthy suitor. It was further claimed that he later told her that he would give her a pill to rid herself of her husband, thus leaving her rich and fancy free. If he had indeed said something like that, he wouldn't have been the first young man to propose a scheme that, on reflection, he didn't really mean. The fact that Harris never confessed to Helen's murder, even in the electric chair, left some people with vague doubts about his guilt. But perhaps he only wanted his family, especially his mother, to never be certain of his guilt. Some people wondered whether the chemist could not have made the mistake which gave the pill its fatal kick? It was possible, of course, if not probable. As he was strapped into the electric chair Harris said calmly, "I'm innocent, absolutely innocent of the crime for which I'm being executed."

His mother fought tirelessly to save him and, when this failed, to retrieve his good name. Two days before the execution she had a special coffin made for him. It carried a metal plate which said: *Murdered May 8, 1893.* And later, when the case was almost forgotten, she published a book called *The Judicial Murder of Carlyle Harris.*

DR. THEODORE DURRANT

If violence occurred with indecent frequency around – and even inside – the Emmanuel Baptist Church in Bartlett Street, San Francisco, it was accepted by the congregation with no more than a sorrowing concern. For, after all, this was rip-roaring Frisco, and these were the days, before the turn of the century, when it was still part of the wild and whoopy west. It had taken a private army of angry citizens, formed into a Vigilante, to cure some of the lusty port's more infamous ills, simply by hanging any villain in sight. But the city would need an earthquake to cleanse it, the righteous said, and the earthquake was still a decade away when two ghastly crimes were committed in the church which are unique in the modern history of religions.

If sin sometimes touched their church, the congregation knew it was symptomatic of the age and the locality, accepted it philosophically, soldiered on, and prayed the harder. At times, too, they could be forgiven if they doubted, if they thought the Lord was inflicting more wrath than He needed on their tiny chapel to test and try them.

For Emmanuel Baptist Church, erected by the rugged pioneers who had reached California by covered waggon in the 1870s, was tested as soon as it was completed. The church, which had a higher spire than most, was struck by lightning. A collection was made in the neighbourhood to repair the damage – and a deacon made off with the repair money.

Then the pastor got into a controversial fury with the editor of a local newspaper over some issue, long since forgotten, and while the editor stormed at the pastor in his editorials, the pastor stormed at the editor in his pulpit.

The editor would come to church, sit in the very front pew and glower sceptically up at the pastor while he sermonised. One day the pastor let out a scream, whipped out a Colts forty-five from his belt, cut loose and blasted the editor to Kingdom Come, thus winning the argument.

But things calmed down and the new pastor, Mr Gibbons, was considered a sobering and enlightening influence on the district.

when two pretty teenage sisters – Blanche and Maude Lamont – arrived to attend the day school there and take an active part in all the church's activities.

This was in the Spring of 1895. The Lamont sisters came from Dillon, Montana, and they were staying with their aunt and uncle, Mr. F. G. Noble for an indefinite period so that Blanche could shake off a mysterious bug which had damaged her health. It was thought a change of air might correct a fault which had left the doctors baffled.

Blanche might have been convalescing but she was no invalid. She made herself active in all directions and was anxious to pass an examination which would enable her to teach younger pupils in the church school.

Blanche was beautiful and perhaps a little more precocious than the other girls, for she attracted the attention of Dr Theodore Durrant, who was a busybody at all the church functions. Durrant had recently reached manhood and was something of a celebrity around the church and school. He was considered the member of the congregation most likely to succeed. He would succeed all right, but not in the way the congregation hoped – and leave marks, stains, on the church which nobody would ever forget.

In actual fact Dr. Durrant wasn't a qualified doctor at the time. He was almost there, however, but the nice people at the church used the title prematurely to give him encouragement and confidence. Dr Durrant would repay them most uniquely for their affection to him.

Any sceptic or cynic would have spotted Durrant immediately as a wrong-un. He was just too good to be true. But the worshippers at Emmanuel were nice naïve people who – a common failing this – thought everybody was as nice as they were. If Durrant wasn't pouring over his medical books, all eager-eyed, he was huffing and puffing around the church making himself useful to a fault. There was Durrant arranging the chairs semicircular for the Mothers' Meeting, hammering home a loose nail in a pew plank, dusting at back of the organ, watering the flowers. If the houses in his street were on fire, Durrant was the type of man who would be helping his neighbours save their homes while his own burnt down. In retrospect the worshippers were to realise that such selflessness hadn't been seen since Jesus Christ.

And all these things Dr. Durrant accomplished without a stain on his neat black jacket, a smear on his powdered cheeks. Nobody could ever remember a hair being out of place on his smarmed down hair. If Durrant worked hard for the Lord, it was, nevertheless, clear that he loved Theodore Durrant the best. Durrant had a sexual problem, a big one at that, but nobody at Emmanuel Church would notice a thing like that. If, during his energetic busy-bodying he paused to help a healthy and well-endowed girl up or down the church porch, fondling her as he did so, people were just too innocent to notice.

He demonstrated by his ghastly crimes that he not only held women responsible for the lust he couldn't control but he also blamed the Emmanuel Baptist Chapel, for, like a triumphant tomcat, he placed his kills within the chapel's doors.

Who should be at the head of the queue and offering a helping hand, therefore, than Dr Durrant when new pupils, Blanche and Maude Lamont, arrived at the chapel and its attending school. He was soon picker-peckering around the new girls, Blanche in particular, offering her his wise counsel, lending her pieces of music for the piano, pens and pencils, rulers and erasers, and books which were guaranteed to improve the mind. The other girls – as teenage girls bursting with life will – gently chided Blanche and referred to Durrant as "Blanche's Beau". But Blanche would answer with a soft "no," and then gave a smile which confirmed her friends' beliefs. It was all good clean fun and no doubt the elderly members of the church winked and talked about wedding bells.

But the truth was completely beyond their imagination.

On April 3, Blanche left the Noble household for school in the normal way. There was nothing unusual in her appearance or in what she carried. She wore her every day clothes – a straw hat with flowers around its shallow rim; a blue gingham gown, and in her purse she had enough money to buy a light mid-day meal and pay for her trolley-car fare. She attended all her classes, including a domestic science class in the afternoon, and at about 3.30 she was seen to put on her coat and leave the building for home.

She never arrived there. Her aunt, Mrs Noble, was only slightly worried, but she assumed Blanche had gone home to tea with a friend nearby the church and she would see her at the service that evening. She went to the church and became more anxious when she couldn't see Blanche among the congregation. She saw young Dr. Durrant who came over to her and waved a book. "Where's Blanche" he asked in surprise.

Mrs. Noble was evasive.

"I thought she would be with you," said the medical student. "She said she would be here and I brought a book she wanted."

After the service, Mrs. Noble avoided the persistent and curious young doctor and hurried home. Still no Blanche. She and her husband spent another sleepless night, and in the morning Mr.

Noble hurried to the school. There he was told that Blanche had been seen leaving presumably for home at about 3.30 on the previous – Wednesday – afternoon.

Inexplicably, the Nobles didn't yet go to the police. They waited through another night and a day. Perhaps they thought Blanche had gone off with a man and hoped she would return, or they might hear from her, and thus avoid a scandal.

When they went to the police, they were asked the usual questtions. Had she been staying out late or away from the house recently? Had there been any problems with boys? The police then asked permission to go through Blanche's belongings and read her letters. But there was nothing in the letters which might explain her absence. A description of Blanche, prepared for the local newspapers, included the fact that she had been wearing three inexpensive rings – one of plain gold with a diamond chip, another similar to this, and a third was a garnet.

The police went to see Minnie Edwards, who was eighteen, who had become Blanche's friend, and who lived near the Nobles. The two girls usually came home on the trolly-car together.

Yes, Minnie and Blanche had left school together on the Wednesday afternoon. They had gone to the trolly stop together – and then a young man had come up and started to flirt with Blanche. When the trolly-car had arrived, Minnie had got on. She had already moved away from Blanche and the young man, she said, sensing that she was in the way.

She had got on the first section of the car and, looking back, she had seen Blanche and the boy get on the second section. She had presumed that the young man was going to take Blanche home. Surprisingly, however, Minnie hadn't looked round when she got off at her stop to see if they were still in the second section. Perhaps she didn't want them to see her look back. She might have been a little jealous, she might have been annoyed, so Minnie sprang from the bus and walked along the street, without looking back.

The detectives asked her if she knew the young man.

`"Why yes," she said. "It was Theodore Durrant. He's stuck on her, you know."

Another two pupils at the school confirmed seeing Durrant and Blanche on the trolly. They reported the young couple as laughing and joking together.

The detectives next called on Dr. Durrant. He was of medium height, had a sallow complexion, was smartly dressed and spoke softly and with respect, frequently calling the police "sir". One of the detectives, Sergeant Anthony, noticed a peculiar shine in his eyes which made them look glazed.

They had heard nothing but good about the medical student in their investigation. He was one of the Baptist Church's hardest workers and most enthusiastic supporters. He was frank and forthright. "Yes, I know Blanche." He said *know*, not *knew*. Tenses have caught more than one murderer.

He laughed when the police repeated the rumours about a romance. "We are just friends with common interests, sir," he said. "I'm still completing my medical studies. I haven't got the time for a serious romance."

But the detectives were surprised by Durrant's answer to their next question. "When did you last see her, doctor?"

Durrant said he couldn't be a hundred per cent sure, but he might have seen her on the Monday or the Tuesday – she disappeared on the Wednesday – but if he hadn't seen her on those two days he had certainly seen her at the services on Sunday.

"But several people saw you on the trolly-car with her on Wednesday shortly after 3.30?"

"Nonsense," said Durrant with a smile. "I couldn't have been there then because I was in classes at the Cooper Medical School until 4.30."

"But you did go to Bartlett Street on Wednesday afternoon?"

"Yes. But later – sometime after four-thirty. I went to see George King, the organist. He's a friend of mine and I knew he would be there, practising. I made myself generally useful."

Durrant dropped an innuendo before the detectives left. "I can't imagine where Blanche is. We weren't really that close, sir, that she would confide details of her private life to me." And then added, "No, I've never seen Blanche with any man or heard her speak of anybody."

The detectives were confused: there were three witnesses who said they'd seen Durrant and Blanche together on Wednesday.

They found yet another witness, a student named Martin Quinlan, who said he had seen Durrant on the trolly-car. "He was with a girl," he said, "but I didn't know who she was."

The story appeared in the newspapers and another witness came forward. She was Mrs. Leak who lived opposite the Emmanuel Church. She was quite specific – she had seen Dr. Durrant go into the church at about four thirty on Wednesday afternoon.

"He wasn't alone. He had a girl with him. I didn't know the girl but she fits the description given in the newspapers. I was looking out for my own daughter at the time."

Mrs. Leak added significantly, "No, I didn't think it odd that a young couple should be going into church at that time of day. There's always something going on over at the Emmanuel. But they didn't go into the church by the main door, but through a side gate in the fence and then through a side door."

She added, "Perhaps that wasn't unusual in itself, but I noticed that she seemed reluctant to go, and he was urging her to come, holding her arm but not actually forcing her."

It looked, if Mrs. Leak was to be believed, as if Durrant had persuaded Blanche to get off the trolly, return to the church with him and maiden modesty was demanding that Blanche put up a token resistance against the force of his masculinity.

The detectives next saw George King, the church organist. Yes, he had seen his friend, Theo Durrant, on Wednesday afternoon. No, he had been alone, no girl was with him, and he thought the time had been later than Mrs. Leak suggested. King thought Durrant had arrived at about four-fifty, which gave him the necessary time to get from the medical school to the Emmanuel Church after leaving classes.

"I was in the room we use for Sunday school," said King. "I was practising the music for the Easter festival. Then I smelt gas and thinking it was coming from the library I unlocked the door and looked in. But I couldn't find a break in the pipe."

Both he and Durrant had been given keys to the library as trusted members of the church. And then King added:

"After that I hadn't played more than a dozen bars when the door burst open and Durrant staggered into the room. His jacket and hat were missing and he looked awful. His face was deathly pale and bathed in sweat, and his hair was in disorder. There was a strange expression on his face which I had never seen before. I was alarmed and asked him if he were ill.

"He said he had been at the top of the church, fitting the electric wires, that the gas was escaping terribly, and that it had almost overcome him. He asked me to get him a bromo-seltzer from the drug-store at the corner of 22nd Street, which I did. We went into the church kitchen, where I mixed it and he drank it. It seemed to revive him and he asked me to help him carry down the organ from the church loft to the vestry. I did so, though it wouldn't be needed until Easter for the children's service. He complained of being tired and said, 'I am all used up on account of that confounded gas.' We left the church together after that. Durrant accompanied me to my own home. He seemed better then."

King added that he had been surprised that the gas had made Durrant so ill. For when he had gone to the loft with him to get the organ it hadn't been powerful enough to make him queasy.

The detectives went to see Dr. Durrant again, and now he

admitted saying it was an oversight, that he had seen Blanche on April 3. But he maintained it was in the morning, on the way to school, and not on the way home in the afternoon. When he met her in the morning he had asked her to come with him to George King's home, but she had declined because she said it would make her late for school. He also denied Mrs Leak's story, declaring that he hadn't arrived at the church at about twenty minutes past four, but about a half hour later. "Nor," he declared, "was there a girl or anybody else with me."

He hadn't seen King on his arrival but had gone to the loft. The gas had affected him badly and he had gone down, found King, who had fetched a powder from the druggist's, which he had then taken and then felt better. He had gone home after leaving King at his front door, arriving there at about 6.30, had eaten his supper and then gone back to the church for the evening service, where he had asked Mrs. Noble where Blanche was.

"I was not," Durrant declared "on the Bartlett Street car at any time that day with Blanche Lamont, and if she visited the church at all that evening it was not with me."

The police, still baffled, went away to re-think and re-examine the evidence and the statements they had, but meanwhile, ever the busy-body, Dr. Durrant, with a smirk here and a wink there, was damaging Blanche's reputation. He had used innuendo again in his second statement to the police – *if she visited the church at all that evening it was not with me*. He didn't have to be so circumspect with Blanche's friends at the church, where her disappearance had caused a sensation. He suggested that Blanche, if the truth came out, would be found hiding somewhere, and she would not be alone.

When he met Mrs. Noble, he poured the poison in that unhappy woman's direction by saying that when he had spoken to Blanche on the Wednesday morning. "She told me: 'I am tired of this humdrum life and I might suddenly throw it all up and go away'."

Mrs. Noble had responded vigorously, "That's not like Blanche."

Durrant had shrugged. "I'm afraid, Mrs Noble, that Blanche is probably unwilling to give up this new life she is leading."

Mrs. Noble discussed the matter with her husband. It made them feel a little better, led them to hope that there might be something in what Durrant said. After all, better a Blanche alive, even if she was living in sin, than a Blanche dead.

San Francisco, a Babylon, was far from Blanche's hick home-town of Dillon. Frisco's colourful nightlife was made to boom by the gold that poured into the port. It had gaming rooms with expensive trappings, restaurants with finer and more varied food than any small-town girl would have ever seen, and nightclubs which gave off a false glamour. There was much which might attract a girl to the Barbary Coast, especially an attractive girl who might have tired of the predictability and drabness of church functions and the lack-lustre and dryness of the men. As the days passed Dr. Durrant, with his customary energy, was active, with a sly wink here, an insinuation there. "It's the sly, shy quiet ones you have to watch," he would say. "I know. I'm a doctor." And, "Only the fact I'm a gentleman and a Christian stops me from telling you where Blanche is now." When he let loose this tit-bit, Dr. Durrant would look in the direction of the Barbary Coast.

Minnie Williams – not to be confused with Minnie Edwards, Blanche's other friend – was quick in defending her missing chum. The fair-haired eighteen-year-old would clench her fists and round on Durrant, angrily defend Blanche and tell the doctor to drop dead. Brave and faithful friend, she would pay for her indiscretion with her life.

Meanwhile, slow-moving and mostly ineffective, the police were visiting Frisco's pawnbrokers. One pawnbroker reported, "Yes, a young man was in here offering three rings which fit the description of those of the missing girl. I didn't like the look of him, somehow, so I refused to accept the pledge."

But the police found another pawnbroker who had taken the rings. A young man had pawned the rings but, unfortunately, a day or so later, he recovered them. The police had a golden opportunity and it should have been as obvious to them as Golden Gate Bridge – but they didn't take it even if they thought about it. They should have taken the pawnbrokers to have a look at Dr. Durrant. They certainly had more reason to doubt him now because they had heard that he was blacking Blanche's character at the Baptist school. One can imagine the reason why they hesitated. The Durrants were prosperous middle class and the lowly lawmen didn't wish to annoy anybody. They were showing perhaps unnecessary delicacy, too, in not searching the Emmanuel Church. Both assignments could have been carried out surreptitiously, the church could have been searched at dawn before anybody was about, and the pawnbrokers could have made casual visits to the Cooper Medical School, where Durrant was training.

One cannot imagine police today – more worldly, if more refined than those Frisco cops of old – not bringing the pawnbroker and Durrant together, and certainly a search of the church, no matter what the congregation might think about it, would be high on their list of assignment priorities.

Easter came and things began to happen. On the evening of Good Friday, another girl vanished. She was Minnie Williams who had been so vigorous in defending Blanche's reputation against the snide insinuations from Dr. Durrant. And, early on Saturday morning, a package arrived at the Noble's home, which held the three rings Blanche had worn when she left home on that fateful Wednesday. The rings were wrapped in newspaper, there was no explanatory note, and the address on the envelope had been printed.

It made the Nobles and sister Maude feel better. Mrs. Noble saw the return of the rings as an indication that Blanche was alive – and began to hope. "It's Blanche's way of telling us she's alive and well," she said. The fact that Blanche hadn't used the opportunity to slip in a brief note didn't make her anxious, for the poor woman was eager to clutch at any straw.

Disillusionment came at lunch-time when the news reached the Nobles that Minnie Williams, close friend of Blanche, had gone – unaccountably – missing.

Like Blanche Lamont, Minnie Williams had been lively and attractive. If the Baptist church had held a beauty competition, significantly, both girls would have been in the finalists. Minnie hadn't been staying with her parents, with whom she had broken. For sometime she had been staying with Mrs. Voy. Dr. Vogel was holding a Young People's Meeting at his home nearby the Emmanuel Church on Friday evening, and Minnie left to go to it. She never got there, and never returned to Mrs. Voy's home.

Dr. Vogel, a church elder, was certain Minnie Williams hadn't arrived at the meeting. Other youngsters confirmed this too. The detectives asked whether Dr. Durrant had been there.

"Yes," said Dr. Vogel. "But he arrived late. He didn't get here until about nine-thirty. We were just thinking of closing down, as a matter of fact. He looked ill, I remember. His features were pale, and he was bathed in sweat. He asked me for permission to go and wash. This I gave. He came back after an interval of a few minutes and he looked remarkably improved. He was smiling and talkative."

Had the killer who needed a Bromo-seltzer after his first murder, needed another powder after his second? Or was he taking something much stronger to bring about such a change? This, nobody will ever know.

Throughout Saturday, the workers at the church discussed the latest sensation. They remembered what Dr. Durrant had said, and they also remembered that Minnie was Blanche's friend.

Both girls were lively and some of them must have wondered if Blanche hadn't found lodgings somewhere in the less salubrious sections of the town and sent word to Minnie.

Several women, discussing the disappearances, made their way to the church library. They were going to fetch vases to hold the extra flowers needed for the Easter Sunday Service. Entering the library, they found Minnie Williams.

She was dead, naked, and had been horribly mutilated by a knife. A reconstruction of the crime showed that she had been killed in a smaller room which led from the library and was rarely used – and then dragged into the library and left spread-eagled on the carpet in the centre of the room like a sacrificial offering. All her clothes had been torn or ripped from her body – and her panties had been forced down her throat with a stick. Blood was everywhere. To add to her death agonies and the mutilations a blunt knife had been used and her body was a cob-web of wounds. Her throat and her arteries and tendons were slashed – and the murder weapon, a final obscenity, had been driven into the girl's breast and left there.

Even the police couldn't miss the implications. The killer was somebody who not only hated women and was a sadist, but also carried a deep resentment against the church. They immediately began a search of the church and the outside buildings. They no longer had any doubt that somewhere in the building they would find Blanche Lamont. The street became thronged with people as night fell, and a guard was left overnight at the doors. There was only one part of the church not yet searched – the unusually high spire – and they would do that at daybreak. They rememb-bered the spire was where Young Durrant had been when he said the smell of gas had made him giddy.

It hadn't been gas which had made him ill but the shock of his crime or, even more probably, the realisation of what would happen to him if he was caught, but, such is the power of Bromo-seltzer, that the young doctor had soon recovered. Detectives had earlier rushed to Durrant's home, and not surprisingly found the young busybody gone, had flown. Durrant's sister told the detectives that they would find the eager young man at Mount Diablo. He had gone there, she thought, to spend a few days with the United States Signal Corps.

Apparently the doctor liked to get away from church activities every now and then. He found them clannish and claustrophobic. The sister thought, of course, that having left everything ship-shape down on Bartlett Street, the indefatigable young man deserved a rest . . . a few days in the brisk fresh air swopping cracks with the sodjer-boys.

His sister was amazed that the detectives wanted to search Durrant's room. But they wouldn't listen to any protests. They found nothing incriminating. Everything, like the hair on the young doctor's head, was neat and tidy. You could have wiped cottonwool across his things and it would have shown up pristine white. Every cushion, hairbrush, book, and what have you, was in a correct place, just like marching soldiers. Nothing was found discreetly hidden away. No dirty books, no saucy photographs. Perhaps that had been the trouble; a highly-strung and basically unstable youth had worked too hard and played too little.

They found the suit of clothes which, his sister confirmed, he had worn on the Friday evening. Close examination revealed no blood but these were elementary days in medical jurisprudence. Since there had been so much blood it is hard to see how Durrant's clothing didn't carry large splashes, and the presumption must be that he stripped off his clothing before attacking the victims with his knife, perhaps knocking her unconscious first.

But the careful young man had erred. Detectives found a purse in the suit and in it they found a clip of ferry tickets for stages between Alameda and Frisco and back – and Minnie had been staying with Mrs. Voy at Alameda.

When dawn came on that Easter Sunday, detectives climbed to the high-peaked spire of Emmanuel Church. They had to go single-file up the circular staircase. If Blanche Lamont had climbed up the stairs with Dr. Durrant, she would have gone first. The presumption had to be that she had gone to the spire willingly.

Willingly but perhaps innocently. Perhaps Dr. Durrant had told her of the fine view of Frisco you could get from the steeple; or perhaps they had reached that point of flirtatious understanding – which Mrs. Leak's testimony suggested they had – and were going to the privacy of the spire, where very few people were likely to interrupt their necking.

Blanche was still in the steeple.

The police had to search about in the bad light for a time before they found her. She had been tucked away with fastidious neatness on a narrow ledge under the eaves – neatly but not comfortably. The killer had been forced to push her hard to get her inside. Her young body had been submitted to the same atrocities as Minnie Williams. It had been gouged and ripped not only by a blunt knife but by fingernails. To confirm that a medical student was the killer her body had been carefully raised, with her head on a block, like a corpse would be raised at a medical school's anatomy lesson. But unlike Minnie, Blanche had not been raped.

146

All Blanche's clothing had been removed and these began to turn up in bits and pieces throughout the day. The killer had hidden them in crannies and cavities around the church, below as well as in the loft.

The only discrepancy was the odd fact that while he had made every attempt to hide Blanche's body, he had acted quite differently in the case of Minnie.

Had he not bothered to hide Minnie because he knew that while he might have got away with the first murder he would never get away with the second? Or had he hidden Blanche because he was fond of her – as many people could testify – and he either knew the crime might be laid against him or because, being fond of her, he didn't want people to see her in her mutilated state? He had no affection for Minnie – who had argued fiercely with him in Blanche's defence. He might have thought, in his twisted mind therefore, that he was dealing more severely with Minnie not only by raping her but leaving her battered corpse obscenely exposed for all to see.

But Dr. Durrant certainly made no attempt to flee. To be sure he had left the city, but the detectives found him heading for Mount Diablo where he had told his sister he was going. The surprised detectives apprehended him just before he reached the mountains, and he showed convincing horror on hearing that the two girls had been raped and brutally murdered in the church. Yes, he would return with the police immediately and help in the matter in any way he could. There was a huge crowd waiting at the ferry landing when Durrant, handcuffed – but every hair in place – was brought off the boat at Frisco.

"Lynch him," they shouted. They waved guns, ropes and fists. Anticipating this, the police had reinforced the area. Their problem to keep Durrant alive until he could be tried and judicially hanged. Durrant was still the whipper-snapper. He indicated the mob and said, "They will remember this day with sorrow. When I am acquitted of this terrible crime, they will be apologetic."

He denied writing a letter to Millie Williams to meet him, but Mrs. Voy said she had seen the letter and Millie told her it was from Durrant. She thought he wanted to see her urgently because he had news of Blanche's whereabouts. Durrant's explanation for the purse was that he had found it on the path outside the home of Dr. Vogel – at the side of the house, he said. His interpretation was that if it had been Millie's Dr Vogel had some explaining to do about the missing girl.

At his trial, his defence counsel had a new suspect. They thought the killer was the pastor, Reverend Gibbons. He had more access than anybody to the church, they maintained, and his behaviour throughout had been strange. They didn't quite specify how the poor old gentleman's behaviour had been strange but the pastor had been looking like a crushed man after the terrible crimes were discovered. Friends wondered how he was supposed to look with two of his charges brutally murdered and their nude bodies left in the church – and one of his star followers facing the gallows for the crime.

The prosecution was hazy on only one point: motive. It was as if, for them, sexual mania was something new and not quite believable and they would have prefered a reason for the murders which ordinary simple men could understand. So the main avenue of their case was that Durrant had murdered Blanche in the spire when she had refused his advances and had killed Minnie because she had defended Blanche against his insinuations. Another link of argument was that she suspected the truth. They threw in, as extra weight, the suspicion that Durrant was a sexual degenerate. But these were early pioneer days.

Durrant was curious to know why his friend, George King, the organist, hadn't been investigated. But if King couldn't satisfactorily account for his movements when Blanche had died, he had witnesses to show he wasn't at the church, and that he was with a crowd of people, when Minnie had been slain.

Durrant still insisted on going onto the witness stand. Nobody remembered a hair being out of place at the trial. Each day he appeared with a fresh pink carnation in the lapel of a freshly-pressed suit.

He fought a verbal duel with the prosecutor, and was, by no means always defeated in arguments, although the testimony was heavy against him. His performance was described as fantastic by the contemporary newspapers. He lied beautifully, calmly and eloquently, and there was always a smug, self-satisfied smile on his lips.

It took the jury only twenty minutes to reach their verdict of guilty but it would be another two years before the baby-faced killer, neatly attired, stepped onto the gallows. It was two years in which his family, believing him innocent, impoverished themselves in their attempts to get a retrial and find fresh evidence.

The police continued their investigation to thwart the attempts of the family to get a retrial, and they found hints of other murders. Many women who had known the doctor had mysteriously vanished. The police were making up for lost time; had they been more prompt in believing witnesses like Minnie Edwards, who had seen Durrant with Blanche at the trolly-stop, they might well have caught the smooth-talking doctor earlier and certainly saved Minnie Williams's life.

Durrant went to the gallows on January 7, 1898. He was smiling and confident, and eloquent to the end – but lying all the way to the grave. He said, in a farewell speech, before officiously signalling the hangman to get on with it:

"If any man thinks I'm going to spring a sensation, I'm not – unless it's a sensation to say I'm an innocent man brought to my death by my persecutors. But I forgive them all. I forgive everyone who has persecuted me, an innocent man, whose hands have never been stained with blood, and I go to meet my God with forgiveness for all men."

More inexplicable than his lies was why this religious young man, having committed such terrible crimes, left the remains at the church he professed to love.

DR. HAWLEY HARVEY CRIPPEN

There could have been no couple more ill-matched in lower middle class London in the 1900s than Dr. and Mrs. Hawley Harvey Crippen. Mrs. Crippen, ebulient and high-breasted, was the sort of person you noticed before she arrived; her husband, the little doctor, the sort of person you never noticed. Like most of the doctors (in this work) who resorted to poison, Dr. Crippen was runt-sized. Additionally, being essentially self-effacing man, he was weak of eyes soft of voice, and so pauce of purpose that he was always one jump away from ruin. Dr. Crippen looked, and was, the type of person who had lost the race before it had started. He sprouted a moustache which wouldn't grow and he had lost most of his hair prematurely. The most remarkable thing about him, it was said, were his eyes, which were prominent; but this was because they were so weak that he had to wear heavily magnified lenses making his orbs look like dolphin eyes.

So gentle by nature was Crippen that people simply refused to believe that he had committed murder, when they heard of his arrest. In keeping with his sensitivity he had been most considerate in his choice of poison-hyoscine – which put the victim into a tranquilized sleep. If his friends, however, were astonished to hear that Crippen was a killer, there was no surprise on hearing that his wife, Cora, was the victim. Cora was formidable, and Cora was noisy. If Cora had been with Custer, there would have been no last stand. If soft spoken Hawley Harvey had never been heard to raise his voice an octave in anger, especially in his wife's presence, she had never been heard to lower her voice, it was said, even in church. Cora, then, was a big-bossomed, noisy, vital and vulgar woman, who was embittered by her lack of success on the stage. This, of course, is Crippen's prejudiced view of his wife. There is another. Cora had many friends who reported her gay and vivacious; undoubtedly she had tired of her lack-lustre husband.

They had met in New York when she was only seventeen. Her real name had been Kunigunde Mackamotski, (a name in which she had shown good sense by changing it to Cora Turner), in order to increase her prospects on the stage and presumably, in the matrimonial stakes. According to Hawley Harvey, in a statement from the condemned cell, she hadn't been so innocently sweet after all when they met, but had been the unhappy mistress of a stove manufacturer.

When Crippen married Cora in New York he was thirty, and it was his second marriage. His first wife had died in Utah – nobody has suggested under suspicious circumstances – and, after leaving their son with his mother in California, he had set out to face the world alone. Hawley Harvey found it a cold and unfriendly place and nothing went right for this timid man. He had been born in Coldwater, Michigan, in 1862, and he had studied medicine in Cleveland, Philadelphia and New York. He had practised in several states without stopping anywhere for any length of time. He seemed to prefer England, perhaps because the rats in the rat race there were less noisy, and he got appointed London manager of the Munyon Medical Company of Philadelphia. Even though his qualifications would not permit him to practice medicine in London, he decided to settle in England. Cora's stage ambitions, from opera to music hall, had no success in America, and very little in England. She did get some music hall work in the U.K., but this was only because there was an entertainers strike going on. Her blacklegging got her verbal abuse from artistes like Marie Lloyd.

Crippen wasn't doing too well, as usual, in business, and Cora's expensive tastes in entertaining her friends and in clothes and jewellery, was a source of constant worry to the doctor. For Cora, the contrast in her husband with all the dashing, handsome men she met on the fringes of the theatre-world was so great that she could hardly find a good word to say to him. She dominated and bullied him most of the time, but had the good sense not to do this frequently in front of company. The doctor also got stuck with most of the menial housework.

In these days, with the emancipation of women, husbands might turn to housework without too much of a groan, but it wasn't so a half century ago, and for Crippen, it must have meant a serious loss of self-respect. At one point he went back to the U.S.A. to explain to his company directors why the London office wasn't paying off, and during his absence Cora had something on – nobody actually said what – with an American comedian named Bruce Miller. Crippen would later say that his wife, on his return, told him about the affair in a gloating manner and repeatedly reminded him of it over the next few years.

Hawley Harvey, in a sudden ambitious burst, went into business for himself as a dentist and producer of dental products. With a partner, he established the Yale Tooth Specialists Company. This didn't do too well either. Some of his activities have been described as near-criminal, but even so his weekly income was never much above £3 a week. It wasn't a handsome income and the couple couldn't afford a servant, (indispensable if you wanted to show you had position), and perhaps that is why Cora rubbed it in by making him do the domestic work. But they did live in some comfort, which was possible in the days when you could get six bottles of whisky for £1, or for the same price twenty packets of 20 cigarettes.

Cora directed the pace on every level, and Crippen was such a nonenity that she even brought his clothes for him, selecting everything from socks to neckties. They eventually moved to a gloomy house in a gloomier street, 39 Hilldrop Crescent in Camden, London.

It was perhaps here that Cora sowed the seeds of her own destruction. She insisted on taking in paying lodgers – only men – and required that it should be only her husband who cleaned their boots, took up their breakfasts and made their beds. Cora, meantimes, reported loudly that she didn't do it for the money but because she liked to be surrounded by interesting people. All the men had been hand-picked by Cora. One of these lodgers would later say of the doctor, in court "Restraint in facing her excitable outbursts was the one and only evidence of firmness in his character."

The predictable happened; as any psychologist will tell you. The worm not only turned but he took on the lethal dimensions of a boa constrictor. The spur seemed to be a threat from Cora that she was about to depart with a secret admirer and that she intended to take the £600 of their joint savings with her when she left. Cora also taunted her husband with his own infidelities. It seems she had discovered, which was true, that the doctor had a girl friend.

Poor Hawley Harvey had to turn to somebody, and it was to sweetly shy and pretty Ethel le Neve. She was in her mid-twenties, and had come to work as Crippen's typist in his Oxford Street office. In Ethel he found security and comfort. She was a quiet, affectionate girl who treated him with respect and listened enthusiastically as he told her of his ambitions.

One can visualise the relationship, the silent glances in the office when other people were there, little memories of the day stored up to laugh about as they walked alone in the park; then, two shadows seated in the dark at some obscure cafe; hands clasping beneath the table; references to *her* (probably they had a pet-name like *The Dragon* for Cora); the endless discussions for plans for his escape, as if he was really held in a cage; plans discussed in whispers which would never come to fruition because he lacked the strength of character. Probably, however, the truth was that Crippen did have the strength to leave. But it could have been the streak of meanness he had within him, a product of his years of insecurity, and he couldn't just let Cora have the £600 in the bank, their other belongings and all the furs and jewellery. He would lose his friends, too, but perhaps that wouldn't have mattered. They were mostly Cora's theatrical crowd in any case. The image, too, might have concerned him, the need for an outward appearance of respectability. Could he face his acquaintances when they knew he had left his wife and was living in sin with the office typist? All these things might have helped hold Crippen back, but certainly the money was an important principle in dictating his future actions.

Apparently Ethel made no attempt to force the issue. Rather than an active doer, she was a sympathetic listener, a follower not a leader. Here they were then, leaderless lovers. She might well have had the character to persuade Crippen to forget the money, but perhaps she had decided that Crippen should, for his self-respect and pride, begin to make decisions for himself. Whatever happened, therefore, must emanate from him.

It was all Cora's fault really. If she was really going to go, and take the money in the bank, then she should go, not hang around the house making sarcastic remarks inbetween her bouts of warnings.

Seemingly, the doctor was telling the truth about these threats because Cora notified the bank in December 1909 that she was withdrawing the £600 and closing the account. But even so Crippen moved so slowly that it took him nearly a month to get to the chemists, Lewis & Burrows. New Oxford Street, and purchase five grains of hyoscin hydrobromide. The chemist asked Crippen to pick it up in two or three days because they didn't have such a large amount in stock, and the polite little doctor obliged. They knew him as Dr. Crippen and had supplied drugs to him before. He casually signed the poison book when he collected it.

In those days the little known drug, hyoscin, was used in hypodermic injections in doses of never more than a hundredth or two-hundredth of a grain. It was used for sedative purposes in cases of meningitis, delirium tremens or mania. There seemed to be a touch of a macabre jest in Crippen putting down Cora with a drug which quietened people who went berserk. And, since he didn't use it for two weeks, one wonders if Crippen would have administered it at all unless hit by another one of Cora's verbal and visual outbursts. You can imagine Crippen watching, waiting, blinking at Cora, through his thick lenses. As long as she behaved herself she would be all right. If not, well, he had the subduer in his pocket.

A retired music hall couple, the Paul Martinettis, had the distinction, which won them envy, of being the last outsiders to see Cora alive and still talking. They came to dinner and whist on January 31. Later there wasn't much that the Martinettis could report about that night. If they hadn't found the Crippens in actual harmony, they certainly couldn't say they were in disharmony.

Cora prattled about her work as treasurer for the Ladies Music Hall Guild, and what she would wear for the Ladies Benevolent Fund Ball, just a few weeks away. Crippen? They couldn't actually remember anything he had said or done but, as always, he had been there, politely fitting into the background somewhere, for Cora, as usual, was on stage all evening.

The couples played whist until one-thirty in the morning. Mr. Martinetti had been ill and it had been Crippen's idea that he come and play to take his mind off other things. Cora liked to be known by her professional name of Belle Elmore in the frenetic world of the Ladies Music Hall Guild, where everybody seemed to do a lot of eating, drinking and gossiping, but little actual stage acting. When the Martinettis left, they called, "No, don't come down, Belle, you'll catch cold." So she waved. Their last sight of her was in the shadows at top of the stairs, with Crippen just behind her.

During the next few days, even weeks, all Crippen's resources of cunning which, on reflection, weren't too great, were called upon; and the little doctor moved with an energetic speed which Munyon's had never noticed. On the day after the whist game he popped in at the Martinettis because, he said, Mr. Martinetti hadn't been well. "How's Belle?" they asked. "Oh, she's all right," he replied. A day later, Crippen pawned his wife's diamond ring plus some earrings for £80. There had been more than the £600 in the bank to lose. And that night, for the first time, Ethel le Neve slept at Hilldrop Crescent. If anybody asked she was to be the housekeeper. Crippen was also writing letters in the first person in Cora's name, although he made no attempt to copy her handwriting. One to the secretary of the Ladies Music Hall Guild, said:

"Dear Miss May: illness of a near relative has called me to America on only a few hours notice, so I must ask you to
154

bring my resignation as treasurer before the meeting today, so a new treasurer can be elected a. once. You will appreciate my haste when I tell you that I have not been to bed – packing all night and getting ready to go. I shall hope to see you again a few months later, but cannot spare a moment to call on you before I go. I wish you everything nice until I return to London again. Now goodbye with love hastily. Yours.

Belle Elmore, per H.H.C."

It may not have been Cora's handwriting, but that was definitely Cora speaking. All the secretary had to do was listen as she read it. Cunningly and cleverly Crippen had got the sound and idiom of his dead wife down on paper. But then he had nothing else to do but listen to her for nearly twenty years.

Mrs. Martinetti, in her busy, bustling rounds, heard about the letter, was a little miffed, and when she next met Crippen, and he didn't mention Cora's trip immediately, she wondered why. Had she annoyed Cora in some way that last night, perhaps by trying to upstage her in the talking? She reproached Crippen for not hastening to tell her about the trip, however, and he apologised, pleading pressure. Throughout the night before Cora's departure, they had both been busy packing her things.

"Packing and crying I suppose?" Mrs. M quipped.
"Oh, we have got past that," grinned Dr. C

Crippen now pawned more of Cora's jewellery, collecting £115. Then he did a daring and stupid thing. It was such a collosal mistake that one wonders how and why he made it, for all his moves until now, twenty days after Cora's disappearance, had been right. But now he took Ethel le Neve to the Ladies Music Hall Benevolent Fund Ball.

For a start, everybody there had been Cora's friends before they even knew Hawley Harvey. Cora and these people had their pretentions and interests in the theatre in common. Crippen, a doctor, never really belonged. For a second thing, Ethel was supposed to be a housekeeper-servant. For a third thing, Crippen had murdered Cora and the last thing he should want to do was attract attention and speculation. But perhaps, a touch of Machiavellian cunning, he thought people would be less suspicious if he was seen escorting another woman. A touch of scandal would divert the gossip away from any deeper probing. People would whisper about it, stroke it, and giggle and speculate about what Cora would do and say when she got back. All right.

Not a bad idea. But there was one fantastic flaw. Ethel was wearing one of Cora's brooches and people recognised it. Instead of giving them a little juicy gossip to prattle about, Crippen had given them the truth. Confirmation for the shrewd women at the Ball came when they saw the way the couple remained glued together throughout the evening. They had interest only in each other. For them, they were the only two people in the hall.

In the first week of March, Ethel gave in her notice at Yale Tooth, and about this time Crippen gave his landlord notice that he was terminating his three-month lease on the house. A little later he had the quit date extended until September.

Meanwhile Crippen, and Cora, had become an important talking point among the Guild ladies. The Martinettis were especially concerned because there had been no letter from Cora from America. It was so unlike the queen-bee not to let her subjects know every move she made. Crippen must have been aware of the crisis he had created in the· Guild. He swung to combat this and to carry through the second part of his plan just before Easter, which came early that year. He rushed off a quick note to the Martinettis to say that he had received shockingly bad news from America. Cora was seriously ill with pleuro-pneumonia. The burning question he must face now, he declared, was whether or not he should speed across the Atlantic to join her at her bedside. Why was it a burning question? The implication was clear. An Atlantic crossing took two weeks, and then just to New York, but Cora was supposedly in California. Would she still be alive by the time he got there, was the implication between the lines?

Just a few days later, Mrs. Martinetti and Mrs. Annie Stratton were leaving a meeting of the Guild when, who should they bump into on the pavement, but Dr. Crippen. If they had been more suspicious, they might have decided he was waiting there to accidentally meet them. Although it wasn't really his world, Crippen seemed to know everything that went on at the Ladies Music Hall Guild, even down to the times of the meetings.

Yes, the news from America was worse. Cora was on the decline. The doctor drew on his own medical knowledge when discussing Cora's chances. "I expect to hear at any moment," he said, "that she has gone." If the worst happens, he told the ladies, he would take a week's holiday in France in an attempt to get over it and lessen the shock.

Sure enough, Cora's death came through at an appropriate time, just when the Easter holiday began. The Martinettis received a telegram from Victoria Station, where Crippen was obviously boarding the boat train for France. It said:

"BELLE DIED YESTERDAY AT SIX O'CLOCK.
PLEASE PHONE ANNIE (Stratton). SHALL BE AWAY
A WEEK."

Crippen, of course, had Ethel with him. And, probably for the
first time in his life, money to burn, as he no longer had to await
handouts from Cora. Here it was then: Crippen had predicted
Cora's death a few days before; said he would take a holiday if it
happened and, appropriately, Cora had died just as the holiday
began. Cora couldn't have died at a better time, and she had
never been so considerate of her henpecked husband before.
The way things seemed to happen in an organised fashion
must have disturbed the Martinettis, if not her other friends.

But Crippen wasn't finished. The more people heard about
her death, the more, he assumed, it would be believed. The
dutiful, obedient husband still, Crippen penned off letters in all
directions telling friends of his loss. He even published news of her
death in an obituary column of the *Era*.

When Crippen got back from his carefree holiday in France
he faced some of Cora's friends. They were suspicious and they
hit him with a series of questions which Crippen had difficulty
in parrying. It transpired that in the discussion he couldn't remember the ship on which Cora had sailed, nor the port from which
she had left and, stranger still, where exactly she had been staying
in the States when she was ill. Crippen, an American, who had
lived in California, could only answer vaguely "in the mountains
of California."

Crippen did say that Cora had been cremated and that her
ashes were being sent to him. When he had had time to think
about it, he could be more specific. In a day or so he was saying
Cora had died at his mother's home in Los Angeles and his son
by his first marriage had been at her bedside. He told friends
not to send flowers or wreaths to Hilldrop Crescent because,
shipping being uncertain, he couldn't be sure when the ashes
would reach him and he would have lots of dead flowers on his
hands before the urn arrived.

Some of the friends were convinced. Crippen was a better
actor than Cora evidently. He certainly seemed calm and didn't
appear to be hiding anything. Nor was he under any noticeable
strain. Daily he went to the office at the usual time, in the evenings
he came back. Ethel was now installed as housekeeper at Hilldrop
Crescent. When he visited, he took Ethel. It was noticed that
Ethel now wore more of Cora's jewellery and furs and this was
thought in rather poor taste.

Even if the attitude of the ladies of the Guild were a little more permissive than elsewhere in London since they had pretentions to the theatre, Crippen's behaviour was still stupid. This was the England of the double standard where a Lord Curzon would throw a housemaid out on the street because she was having an affair with a footman while what the noble lord was doing on the sexual frontiers was permittable. It was also the London where the best-selling home sexual guide maintained that spouses should only make love to beget children, and warned that people who treated sex as a habit like food and drink, would collapse with all sorts of unspecified illnesses as well as being ostracised by their friends. And yet here was Crippen wasting no time in replacing a holidaying wife by a mistress and, on her reported death, flaunting her, instead of mourning Cora for a six-month period.

A Mr. Nash was most scandalised by the doctor's behaviour and, far from satisfied by his story, carried out an investigation in the States, where he had to go on business. In America, he found no record of Cora having arrived, and called at Scotland Yard on his return and reported his suspicions. This was on June 30, after Cora had been dead for five months. This prompted Chief Inspector Walter Dew to call at Hilldrop Crescent. Crippen was at work, so Ethel took him to the Oxford Street office. The detective told the doctor there had been ugly rumours and that he must check them – just a formality; and Crippen was so calm and composed, so ready to assist in every way, so forthcoming that Dew was impressed by him. Crippen took the detective back home and showed him Cora's things.

He also confessed that he had told the friends a pack of lies. "As far as I know," Crippen told the detective, "Cora is still alive. It isn't true that she was cremated in San Francisco or that the ashes were sent to me." Crippen's explanation was that Cora had carried out her threat and ran off with a secret lover. He had lied to save his wife's reputation and his own pride and also so that, eventually, he could regularise his relationship with Ethel, who was comforting him through his bad period. Hazarding a guess, Crippen said he thought his wife was in Chicago with Bruce Miller, the American actor.

Dew looked at the jewellery and clothing Cora had left behind. He searched the house, including the garden and the cellar, no doubt casting an expert eye to see if any mound of earth implied a grave. Dew was satisfied with the doctor's story. But he told him that it would be in his own interest to find Cora so that she could contact her friends and stop the rumours. Dew said he would issue a "missing person" circular on Cora and he helped Crippen draft an advertisement for American newspapers.

Dew reported back to his superiors. He wasn't suspicious. He saw nothing strange in the fact that Cora Crippen had left so many valuables and clothes behind. He had found Crippen forthright and helpful and thought him a timid man who wouldn't frighten the skin from soft-boiled rice. Little did Crippen know it but he had got away with murder. His milk mild manner had convinced one of the Yard's most experienced detectives.

But conscience doth make cowards of most of us and Crippen panicked. It seems he sat at home waiting, waiting for the sound of hoof beats on the road and the heavy tread of policemen's boots on the steps, and he couldn't tolerate the suspense, not even with Ethel at hand to comfort him – though she knew not what he needed comforting against. Within a day Crippen had gone, fled, taking Ethel with him. He became famous almost overnight as the first killer to be caught by wireless-telegraphy.

Dew came looking for Crippen. He was satisfied but he had apparently muddled the information the doctor had given him and wanted to get the dates right for the official record. The inspector called first at the Oxford Street office, because it was nearest to the Yard. Crippen wasn't at his office, nor was he at his home, and nor was Ethel, and now concerned, Dew raced back to Oxford Street and questioned the firm's partner, Dr. Royance.

Royance and the other workers, it now transpired, had found Crippen's behaviour of late a little odd. An assistant told how Crippen had pressed some money on him and ordered him to buy a set of clothes, including shoes, shirts and a necktie, for a fourteen-year-old boy. Dew raced back to the Yard to get a search warrant, cursing Crippen for making a fool of him. Soon, police experts were swarming over the gloomy little house. More trunks of Cora's clothing were unearthed, and yet more jewellery. They dug up the garden and again searched the cellar. Nothing. It wasn't until Dew, armed with a poker, went to work on the brick-floor of the cellar that he began to find evidence – evidence of a sort.

He found several pieces of body, but Crippen had used his medical skills well. The head, the skeleton and the bones were missing, and would never be found. Experts (including an hitherto unknown pathologist named Bernard Spilsbury, who was soon to bring pathology back into respect with judges and jury), worked for three weeks to try and establish that the remains were those of a woman and also of Cora Crippen. The only indication that the remains might be those of a female was the presence of a Hinde hair-curler and the fact that some hair was found which had been dye tinted. It seemed Crippen had worked on the assumption that if the remains couldn't be identified as a woman, and especially of his wife, he would go free.

The closest the experts, initially, could establish a relationship between the remains and Mrs. Crippen was a scarred piece of skin, which might, or might not, have come from a stomach. Friends told them that Cora had an operation scar on her stomach. But they did establish that the remains showed that the person had died by poisoning, by the intake of some 2.7 grains of hyoscin hydrobromide; and by now other detectives had proved that Crippen had bought this drug in large quantities in January. Also with the remains, police found male pyjama trousers and a top which didn't match the trousers. But both sections matched garments found among Crippen's things. Furthermore, they established through the manufacturer's label that Crippen had purchased both sets.

Dew was fiercely criticised, perhaps unjustly, by his superiors for not being wise before the event. It was thought that he should have been more suspicious on his first visit to the house by the fact that Cora Crippen had left so much jewellery and expensive clothing behind. Dew was hammered because of his lack of knowledge of female psychology, for not realising that a woman, before absconding, would pack and take most of her precious belongings. It now seemed inconceivable to the authorities that Cora Crippen would cross the Atlantic in mid-winter without her furs and muff.

While nobody had yet proved the remains were those of Cora, the discovery led to a nation-wide search for Crippen and front-page exposure in the newspapers. The case against him, in the meanwhile, had to be built on conjecture and then attempts made to fashion it into circumstantial evidence. It was surmised that he had thrown Cora's head and bones from the cross-Channel steamer at Easter. If they couldn't, however, establish that the remains were Cora, the experts could medically prove that the pieces of body weren't very old. Certainly they weren't five years old and Crippen had been in Hilldrop Crescent for five years. And, by now, they had shown that the pyjamas in which the remains had been found, were Crippen's, and of recent purchase.

And if the remains weren't Cora, where was Cora? A sister arrived in England from the States to say she was reasonably sure Cora hadn't gone to America. At the trial, the jury would give themselves the benefit of any doubt and because of the scar, the link with Crippen of the pyjamas and the poison, would decide the remains were those of Mrs. Crippen, and find against the doctor. But first Crippen had to be found.

The advance of science was to bring him down, just as it had so many villains in this work. Dew played a hunch as old as time, however. He believed, that like most hunted criminals, Crippen would run for home. The United States was vast, after all, and fitting in there as an American, Crippen would soon be lost. Dew's first move had been to alert all shipping by wireless, and it proved a success.

Then came the dramatic wireless message from a ship on the Atlantic, which sent Chief Inspector Dew and an assistant hurrying to Liverpool to board a faster ship than the S. S. **Montrose,** on which Crippen was suspected of boarding. The alert came from Captain Kendall of the **Montrose,** which had left Antwerp two days earlier. Captain Kendall had noticed almost immediately that two of his passengers were acting in a peculiar way. The passenger list described them as a Mr. Robertson and his son. While a father should have affection for his son, and the son for his father, the pair seemed to display an inordinate amount of affection for each other. They held hands and Mr. Robertson always seemed to be fondling the quiet, slight, dark-haired boy. Perhaps in a more permissive age, one in which homosexual relationships are condoned, Captain Kendall might have shrugged, and gone about his nautical duties. But the captain also observed that the boy's trousers seemed such a bad fit that they had been liberally fastened with safety pins. He also watched them at the dining table, noting that the boy's manners were lady-like and that the father would carry out small duties for the boy in much the way a gentleman would for a lady.

He was digesting all this unusual behaviour when he received a *Wanted for Murder and Mutilation* message from Scotland Yard, in which Crippen was described and in which the suspicion was mentioned that he might be accompanied by a young woman dressed as a boy.

Crippen might have thought that he was using sophisticated cunning in crossing to Antwerp before taking a ship to the States, and on a smaller ship than a liner on the Southampton or Liverpool–New York run would be well away from any hue and cry. But on a smaller ship and with fewer passengers, a captain has more time to notice his guests. Moreover, since he wasn't commanding a busy liner, Captain Kendall had time to peruse the wireless traffic. There was no crowd for Crippen to lose himself in.

It wasn't long, just two days, before Kendall was convinced that the boy was a girl not too convincingly disguised; and all he had to do was wire his suspicions to London.

When *Montrose* was sighted off Father Point, Quebec, Dew was waiting in the pilot boat. He recognised Crippen and Ethel as soon as he stepped aboard the ship with the pilot. The dramatic capture and the fact that the crime was something rare in England, a *crime passionel*, made the case famous. And, as happens in such cases, the little doctor soon had a host of apologists, and the missing Cora detractors. The crime became a topic of heated debate. It was pointed out, by some people, that Cora had given her husband a brutal time, and hadn't he shown her great consideration in his choice of poisons? It was a quick, safe and tranquilising death. Cora, big and bombastic, was soon being contrasted unfavourably with the quiet and affectionate Ethel. But in the final judgement, no excuse can be found for murder – certainly not for a cunning and cowardly murder by poison.

Crippen stood trial at the Old Bailey on October 10, 1910. It was a newsworthy year, which had seen the death of King Edward VII and the Earth passing through the tail of Halley's Comet, yet even so Crippen won most of the headlines. He pleaded not guilty, and was calm and composed throughout the four days of the trial, even though his commonsense must have shown him the evidence, although circumstantial, pointed heavily against him. If the remains couldn't satisfactorily be shown to be his wife, or indeed those of a woman, Crippen had had the poison which had killed that person. Moreover, the house had been in his occupation when the body had been buried in the cellar. There was the piece of skin with the scar tissue and the hair which had been bleached. Then there were the pyjamas in which the pieces of flesh had been found wrapped, and these were proven to be the doctor's. Skill had been needed for the dissection, and Crippen possessed a surgeon's skill.

After his conviction and sentence, Crippen's only concern became for Ethel's safety, for she was soon to stand trial as an accomplice. He left a letter before his execution on November 23, just ten months after he killed his wife. In it he didn't admit his own guilt, but he eloquently defended his mistress. He wrote:

"In this farewell letter to the world, written as I face eternity, I say that Ethel le Neve has loved me as few women love men, and that her innocence of any crime, save that of yielding to the dictates of her heart, is absolute. My last prayer will be that God will protect her and keep her safe from harm and allow her to join me in eternity."

Ethel stood trial but was soon found not guilty.

DR. WALTER WILKINS

Dr. Walter Wilkins, who waged war on the lowly tapeworm in New York, was a curious man. He was gifted in so many ways but something had been left incomplete in the making of the man. He was presentable and had personality, and it was said he could charm a bird from a tree, a girl from her honour, and a heiress from her fortune. He was an excellent physician but his lukewarm ambition never got him beyond the stage of the detection and the destruction – occasionally – of the lowly tapeworm. I say occasionally, for at this base-bottom and elementary medical task he proved so inefficient that he got into trouble with the New York Medical Board, who discovered the muddy-looking liquid he prescribed as a remedy was as lethal for the patient as the *beef* and *pork* tapeworm.

At an early age, self-educated and confident, Walter Wilkins decided he would rather work his wicked will on women than wage weary war on human pain and suffering. Although he was often to be seen examining a female patient in his surgery, people soon got the word that it wasn't an old tapeworm Walter was seeking.

Wilkins had come up the hard way. Born somewhere in California (nobody was sure where) he had educated and fended for himself in the good American classless tradition. For a time he had been a successful salesman but it left him with scars, not character and he murdered two of his three wives – the second committed as he was close to his seventieth birthday. It is thought he had already cast a fast eye on another willing widow.

If Wilkins' rise, but not his crime, was in the finest American tradition, his detection and arrest was in that same tradition of get-up-and-go-free enterprise, for it was a private eye who tirelessly assembled all the uncollected facts and proved the case against him after the local police had admitted they had come up against a blank wall.

The private eye involved was Billy Burns, founder of New York's famous William J. Burns Detective Agency. The murder was already three weeks old and the trial cold when the brisk and bright-eyed Billy Burns took the train from Pennsylvania Station to Long Beach, Long Island, to discuss the mystery with the district attorney of Nassau County.

It was March 1919, the war in Europe was over and the boys were coming home. Detective Burns was a snappy dresser. He looked more like the Saint than Philip Marlowe as he climbed from the train at Long Beach. The District Attorney, Charles Weeks, who met him at the station, wasn't too optimistic. "The damned case is three weeks old, Mr. Burns, and the local knuckleheads have kicked it about so much that there can't be anything left."

On the way to the scene of the murder, the district attorney gave Burns the facts. Mrs. Julia Wilkins had been beaten to death with a ballpeen hammer on the night of February 27. She and her husband, Dr. Wilkins, had just got home and the doctor had been knocked unconscious in the fight but had escaped with only light bruises. The couple had come from their home and office in New York because, the weather being mild for February, they had commuted from Long Beach to New York each day.

Long Beach, a summer resort, had only some 300 occupants in the winter months, and the Wilkinses usually stayed away until the spring, living in their house on West 65th Street, near Central Park. So on the day of the murder – and for many days before – they had left for New York at eight in the morning and returned to Long Beach on a train arriving at six minutes past nine at night.

On the fatal night, the Wilkenses had arrived on this train. The tall, bearded and distinguished looking doctor had been observed leaving the station with his wife Julia. The doctor had been carrying a mackerel which, he had told another commuter-neighbour, a furrier named Mayer, he was going to cook for supper. Apparently the slayer of tapeworms had a deserved reputation as an amateur chef.

Mr. Mayer was to see the doctor some thirty minutes later because their houses adjoined. He would report he heard nothing, no shouts, screams, blows or anything which suggested violence until the door slammed open, and Dr. Wilkins staggered in with his clothes ripped and covered with blood. He said, as he collapsed, that there had been two men in the house who had attacked them. He had been knocked unconscious and when he came round he found Julia – unconscious or dead – in a pool of blood.

Mr. Weeks explained to the detective as they reached the small, ugly house: "For several weeks, up to the time of the murder, we had a rash of burglaries. Nothing much was taken and nobody got hurt. One or two people saw the thieves and they were described as tallish, young, and both of them wore grey caps.''

Dr. Wilkins thought his assailants fitted the description of the two thieves. The ball-peen hammer, of a type used by machinists, was now in the possession of Mr. Weeks. Dr. Wilkins had stated that it wasn't his and he had never seen it before.

Billy Burns reflected, as they reached the house, that there wasn't much to go on. Of course, there had been no more burglaries. It was safe to assume that the burglars were a thousand miles away, and would have had the sense to jettison any goods they had left from the Long Island raids.

The first thing that struck Billy Burns on entering the house was that it smelled like a zoo. The second observation he made – being a fastidious man himself – was that the house was unkempt and dirty. There was dust everywhere but in such amounts it couldn't have accumulated in the three weeks the house had been empty. The exception was the doctor's bedroom. It seemed that Dr. Wilkins had been neat and tidy.

The reason for the zoo-like smell was that Julia loved animals. She had parrots and canaries, she had a monkey and two collie dogs. After the murder, the menagerie had been split up and distributed and cared for by the neighbours.

Burns noted that the Wilkinses slept in different bedrooms. He had noted that the doctor's room was tidy to a fault while Julia's bedroom looked like a junk shop which had just been devastated by Hurricane Harriet.

Burns knew nothing yet about the doctor's lack of professional success and his fixation on the lowly tapeworm, but he was on the look for marital disharmony.

Did the doctor like having these pets all over the place? The district attorney didn't know.

Burns went round chatting to the neighbours, knowing that from the chaff of much gossip a wheat-germ of truth might come. But the neighbours had no juicy gossip or scandal about the Wilkinses. The couple had been married for thirteen years, were happy and seemed content, and had grown together like fruit bushes down the years.

"It looks as if thirteen was their unlucky number?" somebody observed.

"It sure does," Burns reflected thoughtfully.

But the detective did receive confirmation of one fact which might point to marital friction – the doctor was impeccable in his appearance. Every time you saw him he was so well turned out, you thought he was going to a wedding; while Julia, smelling of her pets, always looked as if she had been searching on the floor in an over-stuffed cupboard.

Next day Burns went to look at the murder weapon. He noticed that the hammer's handle had been wrapped in newspaper and tied with twine. Removing these, he saw that the wood of the handle had been fractured and had been reinforced by thin wire of the type used to hang pictures.

The hammer was very old and there was no manufacturer's name.

Burns returned to New York and called on Dr. Wilkins who was at the 65th Street address. He noticed the doctor was tall, well-preserved and lithe-looking considering he was in his sixty-eight year. He had been badly shaken by the tragedy. Burns asked him to tell him what had happened – and the story fitted in every detail with the statement he had made to the district attorney three weeks before. The detective left the house with the belief that the doctor's grief was genuine. But he still didn't like the idea of it being two young men in grey caps caught burglarising the place.

Back went Burns to Long Beach to see more neighbours, and on this occasion he visited the woman, a friend of Julia's, who was caring for the two collies, the Duke and the Duchess. One thing Burns noticed as he approached the house was that the dogs barked furiously as he entered the garden. Was that because he was a stranger? he wondered. Or did they bark when anybody, even people they knew, approached the house?

Here Burns learned some interesting information. Both the doctor and Julia had been married twice before, and Julia had been divorced twice and the doctor once. Julia had been sceptical about marrying Wilkins, not because of any shortcomings she had noticed about him, but because she had already failed in marriage twice. She thought she was inadequate and the holy state wasn't for her.

Burns also discovered that Julia had possessed all the money. Her maiden name had been Klaus, and she had been the daughter of a wealthy German cheese manufacturer who had settled in the States. She had inherited a 100,000 dollars, a massive sum in those pre-inflationary days. There was a polite silence when Burns asked about the doctor's practice. He persisted and discovered that while the doctor was spry for his age he was somewhat work shy. And this surprised Burns. The smartly-dressed doctor, with his distinguished air, had given the detective the impression that he was very much on the ball and had a thriving practice.

The news sent Burns hurrying to Julia Wilkins's lawyer in New

York, who reacted leerily to the detective's request to know the contents of the will. After checking with Weeks to get confirmation that Burns was officially on the case, the lawyer said the reason why he hesitated was because he hadn't yet put the will to the probate court.

Lawyers were notoriously slow in their movements, Burns knew, but what was making this man delay, it came out, was fright. He was afraid of what Dr. Wilkins would say when he discovered that he wouldn't get a cent of Julia's money. It was all earmarked for charities, the greater part being donated to animal trusts. Like a gunner smelling powder-shot Burns sniffed scandal or at least intrigue.

The will hadn't been changed since Julia's second marriage had shattered. When she wed the doctor, she had called on the lawyer but he had advised her against changing the will in her new husband's favour. He hadn't liked Wilkins, and Burns doubted that the doctor had liked him either.

"Julia wasn't well at the time, "said the legal busybody, "and we all thought, being her friends, that he was more interested in Julia's money than in her. I mean, look at it, a medical man with his qualifications, and doing nothing more than chasing down tapeworms."

The lawyer had to admit that Julia had improved in health after the marriage. The doctor, he grudgingly conceded, had been beneficial for her and she had had a new lease of life "Mind you, she wouldn't take all those medicines he prepared for her She didn't believe in the stuff."

Burns turned the conversation back to the tapeworm. The lawyer amplified; "Dr. Wilkins specialises in the detection and destruction of tapeworms, and you don't need much training for that. It was a disgrace, we all thought, because his qualifications were excellent. It was an abuse and a misuse of his powers."

Burns thought that the lawyer was prejudiced for some murky reason of his own, but he had to admit that he probably had a sound point. He wondered if the doctor specialised in the lowly task of tracking down tapeworms because the medical authorities had barred him for doing anything of a more sophisticated nature. He called at the New York Medical Society's offices to see if there was any blots against Wilkins in the register. Sure enough there was. Just prior to his marriage to Julia, the doctor had been in trouble for medical malpractice.

It was the goddam tapeworms again. New Yorkers were always in a hurry and often ate badly refrigerated and insufficiently cooked meat at great speeds, thereby risking infection before dashing back to the rat race. Burns checked the medical books and discovered that any competent mother or wife, by fasting a carrier, by using a worm-killing drug or by purging with a saline drink – could cure a patient of tapeworms caught from badly prepared food. It therefore seemed unlikely that anybody could make a handsome living from setting up as a specialist in the field.

Burns checked the files further. Wilkins had manufactured, bottled and sold as a huckster from the fairground, a run-down store and even the pavement a mud-coloured liquid called the *Wilkins Wonder Worm-remover*. A guarantee printed on the label vouchsafed that money would be returned if the infection wasn't removed.

It transpired that a woman had consumed several bottles of the remedy and, finding she still couldn't get rid of her lodger, had demanded her money back, whereupon she had been impolitely told by the doctor to get lost. She complained to the New York Board of Health, and an inspector, posing as a carrier, had brought a bottle and had it laboratory tested.

Wilkins knew that saline, water containing salts, was a tapeworm's worst enemy, so rather than fill his bottles with straight tap water, he had dragged up buckets of seawater from the Hudson River. Analysis showed that while this germ-infested water from the grimy river might prove lethal to the tapeworm it could, conceivably, finish the drinker off as well.

Burns realised that the purveying of poisoned water was a long way from beating a wife to death with a hammer, but by the same yard stick, two petty thieves who stole from chalets rarely resorted to violence especially as their young legs could have out-run the old couple. He decided to dig into the doctor's past. He back-tracked to the day Wilkins, then aged thirty-five, married Grace Mansfield, a heiress, of Napa Valley, California. Wilkins had been a successful salesman at the time but Grace, persuading him that selling was no profession for a gentleman, put up the fees for him to study medicine in New York, where the couple now set up house.

The trouble began when, after qualifying, Wilkins began his internship at Bellevue Hospital, New York. He was soon examining the nurses and neglecting the patients. There were one or two scandals and a dustcloud of rumours and Grace, deciding she had had enough, returned to California where she divorced her husband. It had been a long time ago, but people still remembered Wilkins. If faulty memory often made the malice against him more malignant, Burns still occasionally managed to get hold of a nugget of fact during his research.

For instance after the divorce, he discovered that the doctor had put up his nameplate in a boarding house on West 38th Street. The house had been owned by a widow, Mrs. Suzanne Kirkland, and the rooms were usually taken by theatrical folk.

Mrs. Kirkland was wealthy, and Wilkins wooed and won her. Immediately he made some changes in the boarding house. Men boarders, he decided, were trouble because they couldn't be controlled, so a notice went up over the door *Girls Only*. And even then Dr. Wilkins interviewed each applicant alone before accepting her. The girls had never lived in a place like it. They had their own very considerate doctor close at hand. Nobody was more the gentleman and more solicitious than their landlord.

Most nights, the stories went, the doctor put Suzanne out with a powerful sleeping pill and then went on his rounds. Some girls complained to the neighbours about the doctor's attentions. A few kept quiet and pretended bafflement. Burns heard the story several times and then a neighbour added, "Of course, he killed her, you know."

"Who killed who?" asked Burns.

"Walter Wilkins killed his wife. Everybody said so at the time."

The Detective was told how Suzanne's health had deteriorated. She had giddy spells and was always vomiting, and one day, after an attack of nausea on their stairs, she tumbled all the way down. After that she was a wreck, and the doctor – claiming it would cure her – made her take cold water baths twice a day. To make the water colder, the doctor had put chunks of ice in the bath with Suzanne.

Burns only believed the story when he found a woman who said she had seen Suzanne in the tub with the ice. At the time she had thought nothing wrong with it because the doctor was qualified and Suzanne was intelligent. Burns checked the death certicate, because Suzanne had died shortly after. He found apoplexy given as the cause of death – a sudden severe stroke – but friends said Suzanne hadn't been old, and hadn't suffered from either blood pressure or a weak heart.

Burns noted the name of the doctor who had signed the certificate and discovered that he was still practising. Although Suzanne had been dead for a generation, the doctor remembered the incident as if it had been yesterday. It was this that intrigued Burns.

The practitioner, with some embarrassment, said, "The reason it stays fresh in my mind is because I feel I shouldn't have signed the certificate. I didn't know Dr. Wilkins and I certainly shouldn't have taken his word."

The doctor told Burns that Wilkins had called him over to sign the death certificate, but when he inspected the body he was astonished to find that Suzanne Wilkins had already been embalmed. Wilkins had agreed that this shouldn't have been done, but blamed a mix-up in the instructions to the morticians. He then added: "They must have thought that because I was a doctor everything would go through smoothly", he told me. "I didn't want to make a lot of fuss as Dr. Wilkins was obviously already shattered by the loss of his wife. In the end I put down apoplexy, which was what he said had killed her, and signed the certificate accordingly."

It was only later that the doctor regretted what he had done.

During this same period Burns was collecting a great deal of gossip and very little fact. There was enough information to assassinate Wilkins's character in court, but nothing, nor was there likely to be, to show he had murdered his third wife. But even though he knew that the answer if there was one could only be found back at Long Island, Burns continued collecting data on the doctor's life.

After he had buried Suzanne, Dr. Wilkins stayed on in the boarding house. He let his practice die while he ran through Suzanne's fortune with a series of fast girls. Some ten years later he was broke again, and it was time to either look for another rich widow or return to medical practice. The doctor found the going hard, his age and perhaps his reputation were against him, and and he was forced to resort once again to *Wilkins Wonder Wormremover* in order to earn a few dollars. The creditors had taken the boarding house from him. It was about this time that he got wind of Julia, a wealthy divorcee, who ran a lodging house on West 65th Street. The doctor, in his best bib and tucker, called round to see if she had a spare room, saying he had always wanted to live close to the park. She had. He stayed.

If the neighbours were to be believed, it took Dr. Wilkins a tidy time to win Julia. She wasn't interested in any more marriages now that she had two failures under her belt. The mailman told Burns one version of the the story. He much admired the way "the doc" had gone about wooing her. Wilkins discovered, for example, that Julia had a nostalgic longing for those old German hymns, and at once he whizzed off and took organ lessons. When he was proficient he plonked down at the wheezy old organ in her parlour and hammered out sweet noises. He was also seen perusing a German cookery book. After that, it was only a matter of time and patience. When they were married, Dr. Wilkins started practising as a tapeworm specialist on the ground floor. Of course a notice went up over the main door of the lodging house, *Sorry. No men.*

If the doctor tiptoed around the house after Julia had gone to bed he must have used thick-soled sponge shoes for his wife never heard him. There was no complaints to any of her friends about infidelity. But perhaps the doctor, in his mid-fifties now, had slowed down in that department and the *No Men* notice was merely a note of nostalgia on his part. However Burns didn't get any real results until he met a patrolman on 65th Street, who had been acquaintanced with the Wilkinses. The policeman, who had the unfortunate name of Crooks, had something gnawing at the back of his mind. He liked the "Doc" so he hated to mention it but Wilkins was interested in talking about true crimes.

He would discuss these in some depth with Crooks when he met him in the street. Crooks, being human, had talked about any contemporary case as if he knew it all from the inside, thus implying he was working on it, or that the detectives in Homicide always rushed to him with any problems they had encountered.

The policeman remembered something the two had once discussed – that when it came to murder, simplicity in the act was essential for success. Complicated timetables and weapons were all right for detective stories, but it was best if a person could be murdered in an ordinary, every day way, especially if it could be made to look like an accident. It was this type of murder, Crooks had told the doctor, that gave detectives their biggest headaches.

What was worrying Crooks was that Dr. Wilkins had been very interested in an old case the patrolman had mentioned. It involved a husband who wanted to get rid of his wife, and he did exactly that when there was an outbreak of burglaries in the district. He struck her down with a hammer, injured himself and tore his clothes. Then he yelled for the neighbours explaining they had been attacked by thieves.

Crooks said, "The case fascinated the doctor and he wanted me to go over the details several times. I had forgotten most of them, but I seemed to remember that the man was caught because he told somebody who told the authorities. He then confessed. Had he kept the truth to himself, I told the doctor, he would have gotten away with it."

Burns was reasonably satisfied now that the doctor had killed his wife, but how could he prove it? All he had was a notebook full of suspicion and a modicum of circumstantial evidence which would be shredded by the defence in court. Concrete and irrefutable facts were needed, and Burns went back to Long Island looking for them.

He told the district attorney all that he had learned, and the lawyer agreed with him that it wasn't sufficient to get a conviction. He was pessimistic about the chances of Wilkins ever being charged with the crime.

"But," said Burns, "he won't get her money, which is why he killed her in the first place."

"Don't be too sure about that," the lawyer answered. "He might contest the will and get the money. I don't see how they can throw him out of the house, since it was his home too, and he'll certainly have that."

"At least we are now sure he did it," said Burns, "and if we look at all the evidence again with that thought in our minds, we might well see something we have missed."

Burns went through all the testimony again and talked once more to the neighbours. Mostly he just encouraged them to gossip while he listened. One man mentioned to him how quiet it was at night now they were no longer disturbed by the barking of Julia Wilkins's two collie dogs.

"They noisy?"

"Hell. They were ding-donging away all the time if anybody other than Julia or the doctor was moving around."

Burns became intrigued and a question formed on his lips. He knew that the neighbour had been home on the night of the crime. Burns also remembered the fury of the dogs when he, a stranger, had approached the house where they had been billeted. He said, "Do you remember if they barked on the night Julia Wilkins was murdered?"

"No, they didn't," said the man. He said it savagely, like an accusation.

"But how can you be sure they didn't bark?"

"Because we didn't hear them, and both my wife and I remembered that when we heard what had happened. The only time the damned things should have barked was when those murderers broke in, but they didn't. And I said to my wife "Isn't that typical? It's like when you need a cop, you can't find one.""

"Did the collies bark when Julia Wilkins or her husband came to the house?"

"They made noises, you know, whimpered with joy, but you wouldn't hear them from where we live."

Burns told Weeks that the dogs hadn't barked because there was nothing for them to bark at. There had been no strangers in or around the Wilkinses home that night.

"Interesting," said Weeks, "but no court's going to accept the evidence of a dog. But, I guess, every little bit helps, and this is going to be a case with lots of little bits in it."

Burns dug up some more of those bits. He searched the house

and the gardens again, with no result, and then he went back to the murder weapon – the hammer. He assumed the newspaper had been wrapped around the handle because the murderer had known that the fingerprints wouldn't show up on newsprint. It was another point against the thieves being the killers. Two petty robbers, probably teenagers going out for an evening's caper, would hardly have anticipated having to commit murder. Burns took the wire off the fractured wooden handle and as he unravelled it, he saw that a small feather was imprisoned beneath the wire. He thought it must have either been stuck to the handle before the wire was put on or it had fluttered down from the air while the wire was being coiled about the handle.

Burns had the feather examined by a bird expert. It was exactly what the detective knew it to be, the feather from a parrot. Julia Wilkins had kept parrots all over the house and unless there was a remarkable coincidence, the wire had been wrapped around the fractured handle in the Wilkinses house.

Burns next noticed a daub of green paint on the handle. He looked around the Wilkenses house and found a section of fence which had been painted with exactly the same colour. It looked fresh. Neighbours confirmed that they had seen Dr. Wilkins paint the fence the previous autumn. Burns was both elated and annoyed, elated because he was making progress, but annoyed because he was uncovering information which the local police should have discovered. Not expecting it to give him any information, Burns next turned to the piece of newspaper which had been wrapped around the handle. Newspapers were printed in their hundreds of thousands each day and Burns wasn't expecting much when he had it identified. But Dr. Wilkins was to be caught by this piece of common, ordinary newsprint.

It hadn't been torn from one of the big city New York dailies. The piece which Dr. Wilkins had used to wrap around the handle of his hammer before striking down his wife was somewhat exclusive. Burns discovered that it came from the Lynbrook *Era*, the local newspaper. Since it was sold mainly by subscription Burns hurried to check to see if the Wilkinses had been a subscriber. He had his first set-back in several days. Not only had they not been subscribers but Burns discovered that the doctor didn't even like it. He wasn't interested in the small-town news the paper carried.

Burns shelved that angle for a time, and chased up some more clues which led him nowhere. Then he heard that the furrier, Mr. Meyer, who had been on the train with the Wilkenses on the fatal night had returned to the Island from a business trip. Mr. Meyer had also been the first man to see Wilkins after the attack when the doctor had come stumbling into his house asking for help.

Burns had him go over the events of that evening with him. Meyer was convinced, he told the detective, that the doctor wasn't faking the robbery in any way; that he really had been hurt and suffering from shock.

"What happened on the train earlier?"

"Nothing happened on the train earlier, Mr. Burns."

"They were the same as usual?"

"The same as usual. They mentioned that they had nearly missed the train because they had gone to get this Spanish mackerel."

"Did the doctor or his wife have an evening newspaper?" Burns asked. He knew that the Lynbrook *Era* could be brought on Pennsylvania Station.

"That they did not. They had to run, you see, to get the train and they didn't have time to buy one."

Burns was convinced that Dr. Wilkins was the murderer and he knew that he had got the day's issue of the *Era* from somewhere and ripped off a piece to wind round the hammer of the handle in order to blur his fingergrints. He persisted. "But how do you know he didn't have a newspaper?"

"Because he said he didn't."

"Just like that, he said he didn't have a newspaper? He made the statement out of the blue without being asked?"

"He didn't have a paper," said the furrier, "because he asked me if I had one. There wasn't enough wrapping around the mackerel, it was thawing and he wanted to put something else around it. I had two newspapers – the evening newspaper I got at the station, and the one I took down from here with me in the morning. I gave him one."

"Which one did you give him?"

"The one I'd read, the *Era*."

Burns left the information that Meyer had given him with the district attorney. Did they now have enough evidence to pick up the doctor and charge him or not? That was the very debatable question.

During this time, Billy Burns had been striving to link Wilkins to the hammer. The doctor had been a handyman and had a shed full of tools, but though the neighbours had seen him working around both the house and the garden they couldn't remember ever seeing him with the ball-peen hammer. The detective canvassed all the stores on Long Island with the hammer. He had no luck. He went next into New York and checked stores in a wide area around where Dr. Wilkins had lived on West 65th Street. Still no luck.

Then he tried something else. It was possible that at sometime or other Wilkins had used the services of a repairman. Burns did some more legwork around the island, and this time he was lucky.

"Sure, I know the doc," said a repairman. "I did some work for him about a year ago."

"Ever seen this hammer before?"

"Sure thing. I've used it. It belongs to Dr. Wilkins. I borrowed it when I did some roof repairs at his place."

"Will you swear to that in court if necessary?"

"I don't see why not."

The detective and the district attorney now went into a huddle. Dr. Wilkins, still in mourning, was at his house on West 65th Street, and they wondered if they had enough to arrest him. It was touch and go but they might get something out of him if they told him what they knew. He might give something away under pressure. He might even confess.

The evidence Burns had accumulated looked sound enough, but Weeks wasn't sure if it was strong enough to convince a jury. They had patrolman Crooks story about the murder which Wilkins's seemed to have duplicated exactly. They had the parrot feather and the green paint which linked the hammer to the doctor's home, along with the testimony of the repairman who remembered using it on the roof. They had Meyer's evidence that he had given the doctor the *Era* to wrap his mackerel in. And they had the fact that the two dogs hadn't barked but, as the district attorney sourly pointed out, "No jury's going to accept the evidence of a couple of dogs."

There was the evidence too, of course, of the doctor's murky background, the fact that his second wife had died in mysterious circumstances and been embalmed before another doctor, required by New York law, had been found to examine her and sign the death certificate.

The case looked good, but they knew it could be better. They decided to arrest Dr. Wilkins anyway and hope he would break down and make a confession.

But the elderly doctor proved a tough adversary. When arrested he ripped into the district attorney and the detective, snarling that he would sue them for every last dollar they had. Not only didn't he not give them the confession they badly needed, but he refused to discuss the matter – not his past, not his second wife, not *Walter Wilkins Wonder Worm-remover*, and certainly not the murder of his wife.

His arrest caused a sensation, and while he was awaiting trial, the fairground people at Coney Island put on a tableau reconstruction of the crime. The doctor promptly sued them from prison for libel and an invasion of his privacy.

Then Dr. Wilkins got a major upset. Julia's will was published and he discovered that she hadn't left him a cent. The murder and cover-up had all been for nothing. The shock broke him, saving the state the expense of trying him he hanged himself in his cell.

Nobody on Long Island, or on West 65th Street for that matter, doubted that when he placed the noose around his neck and jumped off of the bunk in his cell that the right man had died for the murder of Julia Wilkins.

DR. PIERRE BOUGRAT

People who remembered Dr. Pierre Bougrat before his unfortunate marriage talked of his then happy disposition, and of the warmth and bonhomie he had radiated. For them he had then been both romantic and optimistic, the sort of young man who would have preferred it if Shakespeare had given Romeo and Juliet a happy ending. It was true that young Bougrat had served with distinction in the first world war but while this had toughened him and matured him in one sense, it had left him naïve in another. Especially in the matter of women.

Pierre Bougrat came back from the holocaust of such battlefields as Verdun with the rank of captain, plus medals, and a fine record as a doctor in the field. He married an attractive young woman, the daughter of an industrialist, but alas the girl, in hindsight, turned out to be no Juliet and very far from what young Bougrat had imagined a wife would be. Not only did the new Madame Bougrat not like children but she didn't think much of sex. Messy, and funless, according to her. As well as a sharp provincial tongue she had a streak of petit bourgeoisie meanness. If Pierre reflected with a smile that he would like to hear the patter of tiny feet over the stone floors, Madame Bougrat might characteristically have replied, with a sniff, "Then we will hire some Japanese servants – if and when we can afford them."

After the war Bougrat settled in the town of Aix, some ten miles from Marseilles, in the lovely province of Provence. Traditionally this was the coastal resort region of the leisurely rich. If it wasn't exactly the usual Simenon country, the situation Pierre Bougrat eventually found himself in, and the crimes he committed, were reminiscent of the mournful novels about human frailty that the great French master produced.

Even though Bougrat had decided his marriage was a disaster, there were, he thought for a time, compensations. His father-in-law, who greatly admired him, had brought him a lucrative practice, the Provencal sunshine was proverbial and good cooking and cheap wine helped ease life considerably.

Moreover, Bougrat, who had been twenty-eight when the

war ended, worked hard compounding his practice, darting here and there in his small two-seater motorcar. He soon earned the goodwill of the local people. The Bougrats lived in subdued luxury – Madame strictly believed budgeting in a stone house on the reasonably fashionable Rue Lenas. And so with little to do at home, but plenty to keep him sublimating in the surgery, Dr. Bougrat passed several years, until in the winter of 1923, things began to happen to him.

One morning after Bougrat had driven to the thriving port of Marseilles on business he took a stroll into the meaner and narrower streets down by the docks. Most ports were bad, but Marseilles, among seafarers, was considered worse than most. The doctor was fascinated by the gaiety and the colour. He entered a bar and had a drink. Several hours later he found himself seated in the front row of a club which provided its clients with a show of stripped-down lovelies. Bougrat watched fascinated as they danced and cavorted before him. No fool, he soon realised that a very important aspect of life had passed him by and that if he didn't do something soon, it might be too late. After tantalising the audience of seamen and *Apaches* from the stage, the dancers moved among them and accepted drinks and offered invitations, for a fee, to come upstairs. Bougrat went.

Immediately smitten by an accomodating whore, he went again and again. But there were problems with these nocturnal visits to the port. Theıe was the cost, for one; there was his wife and the excuses he must give her for another. In addition he had his reputation to consider, for a man of his professional position couldn't be seen frequenting such dives.

Bougrat forgot the monetary costs for the moment. He had plenty in the bank. The excuses were a problem, but his wife seemed to accept them. The third problem, that of being recognised, he solved in a novel way. He brought the garb of the portside layabouts, the black beret, black poloneck jersey and corduroy trousers of the *Apache*, and on the road between Aix and Marseilles he would stop the car and change his clothes. The possibilities of recognition, blackmail and exposure were now overcome. After coarsening his speech and spattering his conversation with oaths, nobody took any notice of him.

Bougrat made the run to Marseilles several times a week for the next few months until, arriving home one winter's morning, he saw his wife waiting for him.

It soon transpired that Madame Bougrat knew both where he had been and with whom he had been in bed. She had hired a private detective in Marseilles to follow her husband.

178

The detective had telephoned her that evening and given her a full report.

Madame Bougrat told Pierre that she had been thinking the matter over with great care. It was in neither of their interests that they should separate or get a divorce while her father, who was fond of him, remained alive. The old man's health was declining and a breech between them might finish him. She had decided that they should live their separate lives and keep up an appearance of marriage. Pierre accepted. He felt much better now everything was in the open. He could go to Marseilles more often and not have to bother finding excuses for being absent half the night.

The situation remained this way, with the home a potential battlefield, for two years. But then the neighbours began to talk. It was noticed that Pierre was often seen speeding off to Marseilles at nightfall. People abroad in the early hours had seen him coming back from the city. He was rarely on hand to answer emergency calls after surgery hours. Signs of dissipation that showed on his features, unhealthy pallor and bloodshot eyes were remarked upon. Often, these days it was recalled, the doctor was late for morning surgery.

Then Pierre's father-in-law died, and with no further reason to keep up appearances, Madame Bougrat removed herself, with her father's money, to Paris. The defection, which was followed by a divorce, irreparably damaged what was left of Bougrat's practice. His patients had long since drifted to the other doctors in the town.

With a failing practice, and an overdraft in the bank, Bougrat turned even more to the bright lights of the port to escape his cares.

It was while suffering this crush of problems in his surgery one afternoon that his nurse announced the name of a new patient. Bougrat looked up hopefully and told the nurse to hurry her in. She was a wealthy widow named Madame Bernays, and she was the sort of woman, then not uncommon in the French provinces, who advertised her wealth by wearing it. While she listed for the doctor her ailments and her conclusions concerning them, Bougrat seemed to have listed the jewellery she was wearing and to have drawn his own conclusions about their worth. The lady suffered from rheumatism, apparently, and Bougrat, on the spur of the moment, made a fateful decision. He produced a drink which, he said, would solve her problem. It did that. Permanently. If anybody waiting outside the surgery saw Madame Bernay arrive, they never saw her leave.

A few days later a young man called at the surgery. He asked

Dr. Bougrat about his aunt, Madame Bernays. He understood she had left home with the intention of calling on the doctor and had never returned.

Calmly and casually, the doctor checked his records. Ah, yes, he remembered the lady. "I suggested she go and see a colleague in Paris," he said; "and I can only assume she did just that." He gave the young man the name and address but in a few days the nephew was back. He had checked with the doctor in Paris and it appeared that Madame Bernays had never arrived there.

Bougrat gave a nonchalant shrug as if the matter wasn't of great importance. "I rather remember Madame telling me that she also suffered from amnesia. She was rather old, you know. I can only suppose she has wandered off somewhere and she will be back eventually, they usually do come back."

After waiting a few more days, the nephew called on the Aix police. They pushed the matter through to provincial head-quarters in Marseilles. Hundreds of people vanished every year and Commissioner Pierre Robert only gave it a cursory glance, noted amnesia had been mentioned as a possible cause, saw Bougrat's name and Aix, and passed the report along to the Missing Persons Bureau. He forgot the matter for nearly a year.

Then he was visited by a local banker who looked most concerned. The banker said that one of his regular depositors, a man well off, had suddenly vanished. He was old and eccentric, without a family, and the banker was most anxious about him.

"Tell me more about this Monsieur Periot?" said Commissioner Roberts. "What, for example, do you know about his last movements?"

The banker said that the client had said something about visiting Aix, where he had a doctor named Pierre Bougrat.

Bougrat and *Aix*? Something fluttered in the back of Commissioner Robert's mind and he hastened along to the Missing Persons Bureau and went through the files. He saw that Dr. Bougrat had been the last known person to see Madame Bernays alive. Next morning Commissioner Robert drove to Aix.

When he showed Bougrat his identity and told him the reason for his journey, the doctor showed no alarm. "Oh, him, Monsieur Periot . . . I remember him . . . bit of a hypochondriac, I thought." He consulted his files. "Yes, I remember. I told him the cure for his imagined worries was a long sea voyage. Well, well, well . . . if he's missing it could mean he took up my suggestion."

Periot had gone on a sea voyage, as Bougrat well knew. There had been a splash late at night and the grey waters of the Rhone had momentarily parted to receive Periot's dead body.

But even Commissioner Robert, who considered himself a

judge of men, detected nothing wrong in Bougrat. In fact, he was
rather impressed by the doctor's quiet confidence, intelligence,
and the signs of industry he saw about him. On the way in, of
course, he had ruffled a few gossips, and discovered that Bougrat's
wife had deserted and divorced him after coming into her father's
money and was now burning it up in Paris. If anything, Robert
left feeling sympathy and a liking for the doctor. "If Old Periot
shows up," he said as he departed, "you might let me know."

During the next two years, Robert took to calling in on the
doctor whenever he was in the Aix area. They became friends
and would sit together drinking cognac and coffee or wine. More
people vanished during the two years, but then people, for a
variety of reasons not connected with crime, often vanished.
Missing Persons reports crossed Robert's desk. On his calls to
Aix, when drinking with Bougrat he might ask if such and such
or so and so, missing from the Aix region, had been on the
doctor's list of patients. Bougrat would always oblige by running
into the surgery to check when the name rang no bells. In all
cases he reported back that the missing person hadn't been on his
books, nor had he known them socially.

Robert would only nod, light his pipe and reflect that lightning
never seemed to strike more than twice in one place. Commissioner Robert sometimes found himself concerned about the
doctor's appearance and the state of his health. He looked a
little rough at times as if he was burning the candle at more than
one end. This struck the Commissioner as strange since there
wasn't much to keep a man up late at night around the provincial
city of Aix. Before leaving to return to Marseilles, he would tap
Bougrat's shoulder affectionately, and say, "Nice to see you, old
friend. Take it easy now. Don't work too hard."

This always amused Bougrat, who would remind the detective
that people were healthy around Aix, so much so that he had an
unhealthy bank balance to prove it.

Bougrat's active nocturnal habits were already costing him a
pretty franc, for the bordello girls didn't come cheaply, and now
he aggravated his plight by falling badly and madly in love. She
was a petite brunette named Andrea Audibert, a dancer-prostitute
in the Marseilles dockland. She was new to the dives and her
sloe-eyes bespoke an innocence which the doctor only saw in
church on Sundays. He found it most compelling. Andrea was
comparatively naïve, and economic necessity, nothing else, had
brought her to the dockland dives.

After spending one night with Andrea, Bougrat thought he was
in love. He went back for another night to make sure. Then the
agony started for him. He told the girl he loved her and he

couldn't tolerate knowing that she would be in the arms of other men, when not in his. Andrea was impressed. She found Bougrat to be a cut above the usual barroom lounger, and this he confirmed by confessing that he was really a doctor and owned a house and a practice at Aix. He said he wanted Andrea to come and live with him there.

But she pointed out the problem.

Andrea was protected – which meant owned – by an *Apache* pimp named Marius. Marius, they both realised, would demand a high fee for her release. Aix wasn't too far away and if she absconded with Bougrat, Marius might find them. He would certainly become violent and Bougrat was not a knife-carrying *Apache*.

Bougrat was forced to return to Aix with the problem unresolved and with the thought burning in his mind that while he attended to his patients, Andrea would be attending to the carnal wants of the ugly and dirty men who frequented the dives. Eventually he could stand the agony no longer. Getting into his car he drove to Marseilles and found Marius. Yes, Marius was a romantic, he wouldn't stand in the way of true love, and was willing to let Andrea go – for nine thousand francs.

Bougrat tried to get the price reduced, but Marius wouldn't budge and, realising the situation was hopeless, Bougrat sped back to Aix. The further he got away from Marseilles, the more resolved he became that he would raise the money.

It had probably occurred to Dr. Bougrat long before this that the most profitable murder he could commit around Aix, where nobody seemed to keep money and valuables lying around, was that of his old war-time companion Jacques Rumebe. The two men had first met at a battlefield casualty clearing station where Rumebe had arrived with an ugly abdominal wound. Prompt action by Dr. Bougrat in adverse conditions had saved Rumebe's life. Now he was always showing his thanks, much to the doctor's embarrassment and annoyance, but Rumebe only had the one life and was entitled to bore with his gratitude.

Jacques Rumebe was the paymaster at the St. Henri Steel Mills in Aix. The end of the week, Fridays and Saturdays, were hectic days for him, as he had to make up the dockets on the Friday showing the hours the men had worked, and then pay them on the Saturday. Consequently, over the years, Rumebe had adopted the habit of dropping into the surgery on Friday afternoons and getting a clandestine jab before returning to the factory. The jab, presumably morphine, would keep him topped up over the next twenty four hours.

If the idea of felling Jacques and making off with the pay satchel had occurred to the doctor before, he had always rejected it. Friendship was friendship: They had shared the same battle perils and, having saved Jacques life once, Bougrat probably felt in some way strangely paternal towards the small, insignificant man in the tattered suit with its shiny trousers who would drop in through the back door, into the office, each week.

Bougrat already knew Rumebe's weekend routine. On the Friday he would come to the surgery for his clandestine injection – an injection not even his wife knew about, and on the Saturday he would again be in the town's centre, collecting a hundred thousand francs, or thereabouts, for the wage packets.

Bougrat left the surgery on the following Friday before Rumebe arrived. He drove in the direction of the mill and met Rumebe on the road. "Hey, Jacques," he called. "I have an emergency which might keep me away all day. A reluctant infant who doesn't want to come into the world.

"Who can blame him? But, Pierre, what about my injection?"

"Why don't you call at the surgery on your way from the bank tomorrow?"

Rumebe nodded and, unsuspectingly, waved his thanks. It was nice of his old friend to drive to the mill and tell him the surgery was closed. Next morning he slipped into the surgery as usual.

He was carrying the satchel with the wages. He put the bag down, slipped off his jacket and rolled up his sleeve. Bougrat gave him a lethal injection, hid the body and the money temporarily, and then sat down to write an anonymous letter on cheap notepaper. This was the second part of his plan. He addressed the letter to the manager of the mill, saying that Rumebe was having an affair with a Marseilles prostitute, and since he was behaving in an irresponsible manner they had better not trust him with the wage collection in the future.

Some hours later he went down to the main post office in the town to mail the letter, and it was there that he discovered there was a hue and cry out already for the missing cashier. It had been established that Rumebe had called at the bank hours before and had then apparently vanished with a hundred thousand francs in his satchel. Bougrat found people discussing the news excitedly at the cafes. He had to admit he knew Rumebe, of course, because of the war. But he could say he hadn't seen him for some time and, if anybody asked him, he said that Rumebe hadn't been one of his patients.

Bougrat had intended to dump the body in the River Rhone, his traditional burial ground, but police were everywhere, watching all the roads and searching some vehicles. Although it was unlikely anybody would interfere with him, one of the town's doctors, he didn't want to take the chance. Gendarmes would have been moved in from Marseilles and it was always possible that, not knowing him, they might search his car.

Bougrat therefore made a fatal mistake. He placed the body in a disused kitchen cupboard and nailed the door to the jamb. Later, with nine thousand francs from the satchel, he drove to Marseilles, where the *Apache* pimp, Marius, accepted the money without a word and told the doctor where Andrea was. Bougrat collected the girl and drove straight back with her to Aix. He bought her some more conservative clothes *en route* and she reluctantly threw away her cosmetics. For now she was to assume the role of a provincial housekeeper. Whether the doctor would have eventually married the girl for whom he had murdered a friend is problematical. It wasn't a matter of her profession or even whether he loved her or not, but of her class. Andrea might have been comely but she was base born and it showed. In the 1920s a doctor could be ruined for marrying beneath him.

Andrea was now on show at Aix and proved a reliable witness for what happened next. Bougrat hadn't wasted any time. He had gone to collect her on the Saturday he had murdered his friend, and Andrea was up at dawn, like any woman would be in her new home, looking over the house, and especially the kitchen. She thought she would surprise Pierre with an omelette for breakfast and unable to find a slicer for turning the eggs, she tried all the cupboards. She was fumbling with the one holding Rumebe's body when the doctor came down.

"We never use that cupboard," he said casually. "And it's been fastened up. Nothing but a lot of pipes behind the door."

On the Monday, the anonymous letter reached the mill and the rumour, accepted as fact by noon, that Rumebe had gone off with the money and a Marseilles prostitute, was all over town.

But the doctor had other interests. He had told Andrea on the Sunday that it would be a good idea if he celebrated her arrival by having the house decorated, and he would begin on the kitchen. On the Monday he went to find decorators and to select the wallpaper. By mid-week the hangers were busy in the kitchen. Then there came a knock on the door.

Andrea answered it and came face to face with a familiar face.

It belonged to Commissioner Pierre Robert. He looked at Andrea and thought she too was vaguely familiar "Have we met before he asked?" He gave her that hard look that policemen have a tendency to assume unconsciously.

"I don't believe so, monsieur," said Andrea nervously.

"Mmm. I never forget a face. Is the doctor in?"

"Yes, monsieur. Will you come in while I fetch him?"

Before Andrea could find Bougrat the doctor came into the

room. He saw the commissioner and smiled immediately, "Pierre!" he said. "I bet I can guess why you're in Aix. It's that wretched Rumebe business, isn't it?"

The commissioner agreed such was the case. "Did you know him, Pierre?"

Bougrat admitted that he had, but it had been a long time ago and during the war. "I saw him occasionally about the town but I avoided him when I could. You see, he was so grateful to me for saving his life that it was an embarrassment meeting him. I had done no more than any other doctor would have in the circumstances."

"The doctor is very modest," Robert said to Andrea.

"Stay for a drink, commissioner," said the doctor. "I must apologise because the place is in a mess. We have the decorators in. They are working on the kitchen first."

As soon as he could, the detective excused himself. He drove straight back to Marseilles, raking his mind to try and remember where he had seen the girl, whom the doctor hadn't bothered to introduce, before. Her hesitant manner and nervousness told him she was new to the household. Her drab clothing and the fact that Bougrat hadn't given introductions told the detective that she was a servant. But even her severe housekeeper uniform hadn't detracted from the fact that the girl was attractive and had a fine figure.

He dropped in at the Aix gendarmerie before leaving town. "Whose the attractive girl Bougrat's employing around the house – and presumably the bedroom?"

"News to us."

"Then she's probably not a local girl. Bye."

Back at his office, Commissioner Robert decided to put his memory to the test. He had seen Andrea before and he knew she was on the wrong side of the law, because he invariably catalogued in some peculiar way in his mind any face which he thought might brush with the law in the future. Commissioner Robert sent for the files and photographs of all girls in the Marseilles area who had records. There were a lot of them because prostitutes had to be officially checked and periodically examined by doctors. And it was in the file on prostitutes that he came across the photograph and record of Andrea.

She was a comparatively new arrival in the city, having been brought from Paris to double as a dancer and a prostitute. It didn't take Commissioner Robert much longer to trace the connections Andrea had made in Marseilles and to reach the *Apache* Marius. Traditionally these pimps had only one name, but Robert knew all about this particular one. He knew that

Marius wasn't the type of man to release a pretty piece of merchandise without a fight or a fat cash payment. It took him about two days to confirm his suspicions that, since Bougrat was hardly the tough fighting type, he had purchased Andrea's freedom and that the trading price had been a whopping nine thousand francs.

Back to Aix drove the commissioner. He checked the banks, and he discovered that while the doctor's reputation was good, his bank balance was often precariously balanced between the black and the red. There were no reserves. There had been no substantial withdrawals, certainly not to the tune of nine thousand francs. Dr. Bougrat didn't have that sort of money.

Commissioner Robert spent several days in Aix. Meanwhile the search for Rumebe continued. It seemed odd that such an insignificant man, and an amateur thief at that, hadn't made a mistake and been spotted somewhere, because by this time the story had reached the Paris newspapers. Police had combed the dockyards trying to find the prostitute with whom the anonymous letter writer had accused the pay cashier of being involved with.

Now Commissioner Robert got slightly off the right track but it lead him to watch Dr. Bougrat more carefully. He thought that the girl mentioned in the letter might have been Andrea who, having tricked the cashier into the doctor's house, had helped Bougrat murder him. A wrong idea, perhaps, but it kept him heading in the right general direction.

At nights Robert would drive alone around the neighbourhood and he often found himself passing the doctor's house on the Rue Lenas. One night he saw a couple etched in silhouette against the blinds and then the light went out. The doctor and Andrea – obviously passionate lovers – had gone to bed. That gave him time, he reflected, but time to do what? On the spur of the moment, not sure what he expected to find, Commissioner Robert broke into the garage.

The only thing Robert found, hidden under a seat of the car, was a black beret, black jersey, corduroy trousers and a pair of sandals. But it told the commissioner a story. Dr. Bougrat had a Jekyll side which had made him dress like an *Apache* to visit the less salubrious parts of Marseilles. But although Robert had already guessed that the doctor visited the redlight district – or how otherwise had he made the acquaintance of Andrea – these clothes told him much more about his suspect. There must be a dark, secretive, furtive side to the man which made him behave in such a theatrical fashion. It removed any lingering doubts from Robert's mind that he was being unfair and wasting his time with Bougrat.

Robert went back to Marseilles. He remembered Madame Bernays who had vanished after saying she was calling on Bougrat. There was also the eccentric Periot, who was said to have visited the doctor at Aix. The trouble, of course, was proof. Before he could prove anything he had to find a body or bodies. It was too easy to get rid of a corpse, there was the sea, and there was the fast-running Rhone which emptied into it. But then Robert remembered that the decorators had been in the doctor's house at his last visit. It seemed, on reflection, that everything was happening in Aix at once. A cashier had absconded with the week's wages and allegedly a prostitute. The doctor had a known prostitute staying with him as housekeeper, had paid nine thousand francs in cash (which he didn't have) for her freedom, and was also busy with more expense by having his house done-up.

There were too many things going on. Robert went back to Aix.

Having committed burglary once, the commissioner didn't hesitate to commit it twice. He drove around the streets until the lights were out in the Bougrat house, parked his car, and calmly broke into the kitchen. He carefully went round the room playing the beam of a torch on the walls. He was looking for a room or a cupboard, even an alcove, which had been papered over. Eventually he found one. It was while he was feeling down the edges of the doors that he touched something soft and squashy which made him instinctively recoil. Then he flashed the torch on the spot and found several worms busily boring a hole through the wallpaper to get through the door jamb.

Commissioner Robert relaxed. The worms told the full story. Human senses wouldn't detect decaying flesh through the paper and woodwork, but the keener smell of the worms would. Robert found a sharp kitchen instrument, broke the paper and then ripped open the nailed door. Behind it, he found a dead man – presumably Jacques Rumebe. He went straight upstairs to the front bedroom and arrested Dr. Bougrat.

Bougrat stood trial for only one murder, that of the cashier. His version of Jacques Rumebe's death was partially believed and it saved him from the guillotine. He said that he gave his old friend a weekly injection to help him keep his job, which was proving too much for him. On the last occasion, Jacques had begged him to increase the dosage and, inadvertantly, he had given him a fatal overdose. He had panicked, he said, and hidden the body, and had decided that the only thing to do, since he couldn't return it, was keep the money.

Bougrat was lucky, Commissioner Robert thought. Evidence showed that he needed the money because he was desperate to get Andrea away from the brothel. He was obviously in love with the girl, and he didn't have the finances to secure her release. Even if he attempted to raise the money by mortgage on his house, this would have taken more time than Bougrat wished to allow. There were the earlier suspected murders – the missing Madame Bernays, the missing eccentric Periot. Why had Madame Bernays been gone so long without a letter to the nephew of whom she had been fond? Bougrat was undoubtedly lucky to escape first degree murder and the knife.

Andrea wasn't implicated and once released promptly disappeared.

Marius, whose testimony might have proved damaging, for it would reveal the doctor's desperate need for money, wasn't called. In the end Bougrat was sentenced to Devil's Island, the penal colony in the Caribbean for an unspecified period of time. He soon became prison doctor in the settlement and did such good work over the next five years, that he was granted a month's leave in French Guinea. This was in 1935.

History repeated itself, for here he promptly fell in love with a dock-side prostitute named Annette du Bois. In Aix, after his wife had left him, there had been several women who had shown him an interest. But Bougrat seemed to have got a mad theory in his mind. Only whores were passionate and any other woman, especially from a respectable family, would turn out, like his wife, to have an aversion against sex.

Before his time was up, Bougrat and Annette du Bois decided to flee French territory and go to Venezuela. Bougrat was penniless and Annette used her own savings to finance the perilous trip. They reached Venezuela in safety, where they promptly got married. There were vacancies for doctors in Caracas, the couple headed there, and Bougrat soon had a thriving practice. Nobody asked him any questions. He practised without incident for eight years and then in 1944, when he was fifty-three, he was struck down by a mysterious illness. While in a delerium before he died, he kept repeating the name of the River Rhone over and over again.

His tearful wife was baffled by these remarks in the final minutes of his life.

If the widow Madame Bougrat couldn't make sense of them, Commissioner Robert in police headquarters in Marseilles, could and did. When he heard about Bougrat's deathbed mumblings some time later, he nodded briskly, and said, "River Rhone . . . then I guessed right. That was where he discarded Madame Bernays and Monsieur Periot but made the mistake, over confident after escaping twice, of not discarding the cashier Rumebe."

DR. BUCK RUXTON

Conditions for servants might have improved considerably after the First World War, but a servant might have had a right to be suspicious of an employer who called at her front door at 6.30 in the morning – on a Sunday at that – to tell her she could take the day off. The servant was a Mrs. Oxley, and the place was Lancaster, England. The time was September 1935 – and the employer was Dr. Buck Ruxton. He was giving her the day off, he said, because his wife and the maid had decided, unexpectedly, to go off on holiday to Scotland. He added: "But do come in tomorrow just the same." Perhaps the servant was too excited by her good fortune to think much about it at the time – though the doctor's good manners must have raised eyebrows over the tea table later that day – but it would all seem sinisterly significant later when bits of bodies were found scattered over the countryside.

Dr. Ruxton was a Parsee from India. He had been born there in 1899, and he had degrees in both medicine and surgery from London and Bombay universities. The 1935–6 was a great news period. King George V had his Silver Jubilee in May 1935 and died the following January. On the Continent the new dictators, Hitler and Mussolini, had found their confidence and were testing their strengths against the moral paucity of the opposition, with Mussolini invading Abyssinia and Hitler re-occupying the neutralised Rhineland zone. In the United States, even with Al Capone and John Dillinger out of the way, the country was still alarmed by an unprecedented crime wave.

But all these events were to be overshadowed for a time by the activities of the dapper doctor, who would terrorise Britain more than the swaggering dictators, simply by scattering unrecognisable bits of body over a nine-mile radius of country in Moffat, Dumfries, Scotland. Surprisingly, the first mistake Dr. Ruxton made – and after all he had a degree in surgery – was to discover that it was far more complicated and messier than you would think to dismember a couple of bodies. His second mistake was to assume that all his neighbours were as stupid as he thought them to be.

Both mistakes were to lend macabre touches of comedy to the gruesome events.

Dr. Ruxton came to live in Lancaster with his common law wife, Isabella, in 1930. He already had a legal wife in India, so he married her by the Scottish law of Declaration. They had three children and his practice was conducted from their house at 2 Dalton Square. It was an unhappy marriage most of the time. Both had quick tempers and they existed in an atmosphere of highly charged emotion. Dr. Ruxton was excitable and could burst into tears at the drop of an insult. The principle reason for the quarrels was his belief – imagined – that Isabella was carrying on with all and sundry. The milkman, it was said, only had to dally a moment longer than necessary on the doorstep for the doctor to appear with unspoken accusation on his features.

The doctor himself summed up the stormy relationship after his arrest by saying, "We were the kind of people who couldn't live with each other – and yet couldn't exist without each other. Who loves most chastises the most." But if the doctor could be forgiven for stabbing his wife while in the middle of a violent argument, he cannot be forgiven for killing the maid, Mary Rogerson also, nor for cutting up and mutilating their bodies and scattering them over the countryside.

Dr. Ruxton murdered his wife late on Saturday night, 14 September. She had borrowed her husband's Hillman Minx, driven to Blackpool, where she had met her two sisters, and together they had walked the promenade to admire the town's famous illuminations. She had returned home sometime after midnight, where presumably she had been met by an outraged husband who had accused her of being off somewhere with another man. Mary Rogerson, aged 20, brought into the room by the screaming and seeing her mistress dead or dying, had next been killed. The three children, although asleep in the house, hadn't been disturbed by the commotion, nor by the doctor's nocturnal activity, which extended well into Sunday, of rendering the bodies down to small pieces. But the chore proved to be messier and more arduous than the doctor expected and he had not finished at daybreak.

He remembered now that Mrs. Oxley was due at seven and raced out of the house shortly after six to tell her that she could have the day off because his wife and the maid had motored to Scotland. Then Dr. Ruxton rushed back home to make the place look reasonably presentable before the three children, aged from seven down, got up to play. Somehow he managed. He got them up, gave them breakfast, put them in the garden, and went on with his dismembering. But there were other interruptions.

Mrs. Oxley would testify that Ruxton, although unshaven, looked reasonably composed, and other callers to 2 Dalton Square that morning got much the same impression, although they said he only partially opened the door to them. To each caller he said that his wife and the maid had gone to Edinburgh, and to a patient who called for surgery, he asked to return next day, saying, when the patient protested that it would mean the loss of a day's work: "We are busy taking up the carpets for the decorators who are coming tomorrow. Look at my hands – see how dirty they are."

At 11-30, the doctor decided that the children were too much to cope with while he had two bodies to hide, and he took them to a Morecambe dentist named Anderson and asked him and his wife to mind them. The Andersons, assuming there had been another fight and Isabella had left, agreed to mind the children. They also saw that his right hand was bandaged (he said he had cut it on a tin-opener).

After spending several more hours alone at home, Dr. Ruxton called on a patient named Mrs. Hampshire who also did house cleaning. He showed her his bandaged hand and said the house was in a mess because it was being prepared for decorators, and could she come round immediately and clean the staircase. He said his wife was on holiday in Blackpool and that the maid was on a separate holiday elsewhere.

Mixing up his stories was one mistake and in allowing Mrs. Hampshire to see the house, Dr. Ruxton made another, for what she saw in the next few hours made her the most telling of the Crown witnesses arraigned against him at his trial in Manchester. The mental pressure of the murders coupled with the sheer physical exhaustion of reducing the bodies to a hundred pieces had made him such a wreck, it seems, that he couldn't, for a time, calculate properly. This is the only way to explain why he made no attempt to hide the fantastic chaos in the home from Mrs. Hampshire after going to such extraordinary lengths to render the bodies into nothing. Perhaps he chose Mrs. Hampshire instead of Mrs. Oxley because she wasn't as familiar with the household. Perhaps, again, it might have been because Mrs. Hampshire was the less discerning of the two.

But she was shocked by what she saw at 2 Dalton Square. The radio was blaring out loudly, and the chaos in the house was indescribable. Plaster and wallpaper had been stripped from the walls, and carpets had been pulled up, and straw had been scattered over the floors. Pools of water were in all the rooms and the carpets were sodden as if there had been a pipe burst.

A meal had been laid for two in the dining room and the food was now cold. There was more chaos to greet Mrs. Hampshire when she got upstairs, where she found doors locked (the doctor saying he didn't have the keys). The bathroom in particular was in a filthy mess. The tub was discoloured a sort of "dirty yellow" to within a few inches of the top. On the linoleum she found what appeared to be blood which had been inefficiently mopped up.

Complaining while she worked, Mrs. Hampshire did her best. She would tell the court, "I gave the bath a good scrub with hot water and Vim, but I couldn't get the stains off." The doctor gave her one of his suits which, he suggested, might do her husband a turn. It was badly stained but the doctor thought it would look like new when it had been cleaned (he asked for it's return the following day). He also gave her some carpets, but when she later attempted to clean these by throwing buckets of water over them the colour of the water ran off looking like blood.

Mrs. Hampshire, however, didn't seem at all suspicious by the mess in the Ruxton household. She neither appeared to ask for an explanation – nor did Ruxton volunteer one other than to say things were being pulled up and taken apart for the decorators.

The regular cleaner, Mrs. Oxley, would have realised something was wrong because she was at the house daily and knew it was kept tidy. But Mrs. Hampshire must have, contemptuously, thought the bulk of the mess had been caused by Isabella Ruxton's dirty household habits. Not satisfied with killing his wife, Dr. Ruxton was also irreparably damaging her good reputation.

On the Monday, Dr. Ruxton hired an Austin car, and on the Tuesday, on his way back from Scotland, he was involved in a minor incident with a cyclist, and police at Kendal in the Lake District recorded the accident. Dr. Ruxton told them he was on his way home from Carlisle after a business trip. In actual fact he had taken the main Edinburgh–Carlisle road until he got to deserted countryside around Moffat, and then began to jettison pieces of body and bone wrapped in brown paper, newspaper and pieces of sheeting and clothing. It took him some time since he preferred discarding the remains into rivers and ravines rather than on open grassland. There were some hundred pieces and four or five pieces usually were put into one packet. The important parts were dumped into an especially deep ravine, and these consisted of several brown paper parcels which included two heads, two legs, two arms, two hands, four or five large bones and a miscellaneous collection of smaller items, including large pieces of flesh.

The discovery of the first packages in the deep ravine led to a search of the countryside and further parcels were picked up across a radius of nine miles. They were taken to Edinburgh University's medical college where experts gathered to try and put the hundred pieces back together again.

This side of the investigation was to prove impossible. The surgeons soon realised that the bodies had been taken apart by an expert. Anything which might identify one of them – like an operation scar – had been removed. Mary Rogerson had a squint in one of her eyes and the eyes of the younger woman had been removed. So had Isabella's legs which were slightly irregular in shape – they had been reduced to nothing. The surgeons came to the erroneous conclusion that the bodies were that of a man and a woman. Since all the hair had been removed and much of the skin peeled off, there was nothing for the surgeons to work with.

It was a jubiliant Dr. Ruxton who read out the fact that the Moffat remains were that of a man and a woman to Mrs. Oxley – "It's a man and woman," he crowed. "So you can see it's not our missing two."

"I should hope not!" sniffed Mrs. Oxley.

The country had been electrified by the news of the finding of the remains. There had been a spate of dismembered bodies found in Britain recently – dotted about at places as far apart as Brighton, Brentford, Kings Cross Station, and found on a train bound for Waterloo Station. It was feared that a dissecting Jack the Ripper was on the rampage.

If the authorities were thwarted by the cunningly scientific dismemberment of the bodies, they had other avenues to follow, and the materials used to wrap up the remains looked like proving most promising. In the meantime Dr. Ruxton could be seen hurrying about his home town looking dishevelled and not unlike somebody who was a day behind in his sleep. He was soon telling contradictory stories about the absence of his wife and the maid. To one neighbour he said his wife had left him for good, to another that she was on holiday and had their car with her – and later the doctor was seen driving the car. To another he said Mary Rogerson was either on holiday with his wife or somewhere by herself. Later still he maintained that Mary was pregnant and had gone off with a secret lover. And soon, just a day or two before his arrest, he said that both women had been deceiving him and that Mary had connived at Isabella's adultery and shared lovers with her.

After dumping the bodies across the Scottish wastelands, the doctor returned to Dalton Square and promptly hired two more

charwomen – Mrs. Smith and Mrs. Curwen– to go over the house
again. They were to report that as soon as they got rid of one
lot of bloodstains, they found more. They seemed to come up
from under the floorboards and from every undetectable nook
and cranny. Soon they were complaining about an obnoxious
smell and Dr. Ruxton efficiently dealt with this by sending one
of them for eau-de-Cologne and syringe, to spray the rooms.

The medical examination of the remains was hopeless. The
surgeons couldn't even get a fingerprint because the fingers had
been skinned and fingers, thumbs and toes had been detached at
each joint. Nor could dental work be re-assembled, for Dr.
Ruxton had anticipated that the experts would concentrate on
this. All the police had after a week of exhaustive investigation
was the firm fact that the bodies had been dumped from a car
between September 15 and 19. They could be sure of the date
because of the state of the parcels found in a stream called the
Linn. There had been a heavy storm on the 18th and flood water
had carried the parcels for some way until the water level had
fallen and left the packages high on the bank. They had a date –
the 19th – on a newspaper used in the wrapping and while
several newspapers had been used, 19th was the last date.

The police, of course, concentrated on the material used for the
wrapping. At first it didn't seem much to work with – a green
blouse, a man's vest, pieces of sheeting and wool, a child's
rompers and old national newspapers which circulated right
across the country. But the police studied each item minutely
and one newspaper, the *Sunday Graphic*, seemed to carry an
undue amount of local news about the Lancaster and Morecambe
area.

They showed it to a journalist who confirmed that the local
items didn't merit national interest and suggested the newspaper
must be a copy of a "slip" edition produced specifically for the
Lancaster and Morecambe area, a common practise with
newspapers when wishing to build circulation in certain areas.
A check with the office of the *Sunday Graphic* brought immediate
confirmation of this fact. It was a big step forward. The police
decided they should look for a surgeon or a butcher who either
lived in or had visited the Lancaster and Morcambe areas on the
day the newspaper had been published. The Lancaster police
were informed and they checked their missing persons files.

By now Dr. Ruxton's first flush of success with the announcement that the remains were possibly those of a man and a woman,
had begun to abate. He saw other problems looming. He knew
that the absence of the two women couldn't go on indefinitely
without awkward questions being asked. The sisters would be

asking about Isabella; and the Rogersons would be anxious because they hadn't heard from their daughter. People were not too inquisitive at the moment because the women had only been gone some two weeks and it was believed they were on holiday. But people will talk and his neighbours had been comparing the stories the doctor had told them to explain Isabella and Mary's absence. Also, the children wanted to know why Mummy hadn't written them or sent them a card after being away so long.

After giving the matter much thought, the doctor decided to change his strategy. He decided to anticipate everybody else by being the first person to show concern. Overnight he switched. He dropped his nonchalant air and began to tell anybody who would listen that he was most anxious about the non-appearance of Isabella. "If she is angry with me," he would say, "why can't she write to the children?" In keeping with this new stance, he wrote to his wife's sister on October 7:

> "I am heartbroken and half mad . . . Isabella has again left me. She has done this trick again after about ten months. Do you remember she left me bag and baggage last November? The children are asking for her daily and I really cannot sleep without her . . . Mine is only the temper, but in my heart she is all."

This was a letter that Ruxton was sure would be passed to the police and the sister would have to confirm that Isabella had left him for a time ten months before – although then, as almost any sister would do, she had kept in touch either by visit or letter with her family. Next, obviously, in keeping with his new anxiety, he must call on Mary's parents.

"Look," he told them, "I'm most anxious about Mrs Ruxton. I haven't heard from her and it's been three weeks. I assume Mary's with her, what does she say in her letters?" Now the Rogersons told him of their concern for they hadn't had even a card from Mary and it was so unlike her not to show them consideration. Before he left, Dr. Ruxton told them it was very odd and he had decided he had better see the police.

It became a race in a sense who would reach police headquarters first, Ruxton or the Rogersons, but the Rogersons won, possibly because their anxiety was genuine. When Ruxton arrived he told the police about his marital problems and asked that discreet inquiries be made into his wife's whereabouts. "I don't want to know who she is living with, but just that she is safe. And she should make some attempt to see the children."

The doctor's assessment of Isabella's morals didn't sit square with what the police discovered about her character from her friends and relatives, but since there was always a first time and Isabella might have been driven off by Ruxton's fiery temper to seek somebody else's protection, the police had to investigate with care. They did discover that Ruxton, on occasion, had threatened his wife with knives and in one instance with a revolver. In fact their own books showed them that on several occasions the fights in the Ruxton home had been so violent that police had been sent there.

The reporters were in Lancaster in force because of the slip edition of the *Sunday Graphic*, and they were the first to link the remains found at Moffat with the two missing women, although they had nothing more to go on other than coincidence and the fact that Ruxton was a surgeon. But Ruxton saw the writing on the wall – the materials used in wrapping the remains was on the way from Dumfries.

Ruxton took fright when he saw the morning newspapers speculating on a connection between the grisly remains at Moffat and the two missing women – one of whom was the wife of a doctor who was also a surgeon. He raced off to police head-quarters to protest, but was politely told that they had no control over the press. However, as he was here, they had a question for him to answer: "Why had he put it about that Mary Rogerson was pregnant?"

"Because she was."

"How could you be sure? Did you examine her?"

"No, but I could see it by her eyes and there were other signs only a doctor would notice."

"He would need to be a remarkable doctor."

"I am."

Ruxton next ran off to see Mrs. Hampshire, who had helped him clean up the house on that fatal Sunday. His concern was the bloodstained suit. As if she was a co-conspirator, he told her, "Do something about it . . . get it out of the way . . . burn it." She would later testify that he was extremely agitated and, remembering the bloodstained carpets, he wanted her to destroy those as well. He said, before leaving her, that he was going to give a statement to the police and asked her not to see them until he had.

The newspapers increased the tempo next morning, and he raced off with a newspaper to the police again, and accused them of being in a conspiracy with the reporters against him. "Why do they accuse me of the Moffat murder?" he demanded. "Somebody will shortly be putting a dead body on my doorstep and I will be accused of killing it."

Ruxton next called on the Rogersons and asked them how

many teeth Mary had had extracted and when the dental surgery had been carried out. He really wanted to know, however, if the police had connected Mary with the remains found at Moffat. The Rogersons said that to their knowledge they had not. Ruxton hurried back to the police with the late edition of an evening newspaper, "You really must stop these people," he screamed. "Look at this – this reporter says that this woman has a full set of teeth in the lower jaw and I know from my own knowledge that Mary has at least four teeth missing." On this occasion he became hysterical and raved incoherently against the police and claimed they were tapping his telephone.

Mrs. Rogerson was shown the green blouse. She recognised it by a patch under the arm – recognised it because she had carried out the repair herself. The rompers, she thought, were like a pair given to Mary for the Ruxton children by a Mrs. Holme. Mrs. Holme was tracked down and immediately recognised the rompers and said she would swear she had given them to the maid for the Ruxton children. The police had three items linking the Moffat remains with the two missing women, but was it sufficient to prove that the bodies were those of Isabella Ruxton and Mary Rogerson? And if this could be established with any degree of satisfaction, was this sufficient to bring a murder charge against Dr. Ruxton? It didn't, on the face of it, seem so . . . unless the doctor blundered in the answers he gave or, his conscience exerting itself, he confessed.

Mrs. Hampshire, and witnesses like her, were coming forward with what they knew and it seemed that the authorities would be successful in securing a conviction on circumstantial evidence – but only if they could prove that the remains were those of Isabella and Mary. A paragraph in Halsbury's *Laws of England* had them worried for a time. It stipulates:

> "Where no body or part of a body has been found, which is proved to be that of the person alleged to have been killed, the accused person should not be convicted of either murder or manslaughter unless there is evidence either of the killing or of the death of the person alleged to have been killed. In the absence of such evidence, there is no onus upon the prisoner to account for the disappearance or non-production of the person alleged to have been killed."

On October 12, the police interrogated Ruxton. He was asked to account for his movements between September 14 and 30, and he replied, "I shall be only too pleased to tell you all I possibly can." He produced a document he had already prepared, which was called *My Movements*, and he also made a long statement which was a reiteration of his declared innocence.

It was decided to take a chance and charge Ruxton, and he was held on remand until November 5 while the experts in Edinburgh put the hundred pieces of bodies together in what was a nightmare jigsaw puzzle. It was a stupendous task conducted by the leading pathologists of the day and among those participating were Professor John Glaister, Professor of Forensic Medicine at Glasgow University; Professor Sydney Smith, Professor of Forensic Medicine at Edinburgh University; and Professor J. C. Brash, Professor of Anatomy at Edinburgh University. Life-sized photographs of the alleged victims heads were super-imposed over pictures of the skulls, and were found to match. Mainly because of this new evidence Ruxton, who had been charged only with Mary Rogerson's murder – because of the green blouse and the rompers – was now charged, on December 13, with the murder of his wife. Lest the evidence not be con-sidered enough, artificial teeth were fitted into the mouths of the skulls to get an impression of what the mouths had looked like. In all, twenty sets of 250 pictures were completed – many taken from overhead scaffolding with the cameras pointed down on the bodies assembled below.

Dr. Ruxton pleaded not guilty when he stood trial to the murder of his wife – and, by inference, the maid. He answered, "This is absolute bunkum with a capital B". He maintained in *My Movements*, which was produced in court, that Isabella and Mary had left for Edinburgh at about 9-30 on Sunday morning, Isabella shouting as she went through the door – "Toodlehoo, Pa. There is a cup of tea on the hall table for you."

But the wealth of medical evidence showing that the remains were those of Isabella and Mary was overwhelming. In his summing up, Mr. Justice Singleton spoke of the medical work done in the highest terms as a "distinguished body of evidence." Ruxton was found guilty and was sentenced to death. Unknown to the court he had already confessed the murders in an article written for a newspaper. This was sealed in an envelope, only to be opened if he was found guilty. It was published several days after his execution at Strangeways Prison, Manchester, on May 12, 1936. In it the sometimes smooth and sometimes tem-peramentally erratic doctor wrote: "I killed Mrs. Ruxton in a fit of temper. I thought she had been with a man. I was mad at the time. Mary Rogerson was present so I had to kill her too."

DR. MORRIS BOLBER

What can a faith healer do to turn a crust when his patients have lost their belief in him ? Dr. Morris Bolber, who practised medicine in Philadelphia, Pennsylvania, in the depressed 1930s, found himself facing this stark reality of medical life one winter's day, and rather than move his shingle to a more friendly city or join the soup queues, he decided to start murdering his patients for *profit*.

It really wasn't so much that Dr. Bolber's patients had lost faith in him as that life seemed to have lost faith with them. They were mostly poor Italians from the Italian ghetto of the Friendly City. They were so hard up, in fact, that they couldn't afford to be ill. In an attempt to make his surgery on Ninth and Moyamensing pay, Dr. Bolber had already been forced to eschew conventional medicine for faith healing, because that was what the superstitious and illiterate Mediterreanians preferred. He had taken on other sidelines as well, much like a salesman would. A little drug-peddling here, an abortion there; and the gangsters already knew where you could get a bullet-hole plugged up or a knife-cut stitched.

Little Doc Bolber wasn't lacking in enterprise or imagination, and he devised other wrinkles to help speed dollars to his bank. If women came complaining that their menfolk were too energetic in bed, Dr. Bolber had the remedy; beer spiked with saltpeter was guaranteed to slow even a bull down. If, on the other hand, it was a complaint of husbandly indifference, why, Dr. Bolber also had the remedy for that, it was a little something, (and don't dare ask me what it is) to stiffen things up. If that didn't work, Dr. Bolber had another wrinkle, but more of that a little later.

By such activities, the doctor had weathered the Depression and by February 1932, when he was forty-two, he could compliment himself on having survived the worst. If it wasn't time for a big splash, at least it was time to relax a little. There was a bit in the bank, after all, and he wasn't in debt. Bolber was thinking along these lines then, when on a February morning, an attractive woman came calling. She was the thirty-year-old wife of Anthony Giscobbe, who owned a grocery store. Her complaint was that her husband, Tony, was neglecting both her and the business for another broad and booze. Dr. Bolber's remedy, a new dress and hairdo for her, and some aphrodisiac pills with which to spike her husband's wine at supper.

Mrs. Giscobbe was back within the fortnight, more distraught than ever. The dope had worked only too well. After supper each night, Tony left the home so quickly (presumably to go to the other woman) that he hardly paused to give her a reasonable excuse. Dr. Bolber, like many a doctor with more conventional medicine, promptly reversed the treatment. He now recommended beer spiked with saltpeter in order to slow Tony down in the evenings.

When Bolber had an attractive patient, he had the habit of letting them talk on, and lonely Mrs. Giscobbe welcomed a sympathetic ear. He heard therefore about the difficulties the Giscobbes were having in keeping up the payments on a hefty life insurance policy that Tony had thought he should take out, for the slump was hitting the profits from the store and, in any case, Tony himself was neglecting his business.

Bolber thought that if Tony was dead, then the insurance wouldn't have to be paid (which was one way of solving the problem), and then Mrs. Giscobbe asked the doctor who the charming Italian was who was waiting to see him outside. The doctor didn't know, but he took a look. As he came back, ideas began to blaze through his mind. "That's my tailor Paul Petrillo. You must have seen him about. Has a store down the street."

Of course Mrs. Giscobbe had seen the tailor and, realising this, the doctor gave it more thought. There was an understanding between Petrillo and the doctor which enabled the doctor to kill a couple of hefty birds with one rotten stone. Petrillo was a womaniser and in exchange for a regular supply of free suits, Bolber would introduce this lecher to his more attractive patients; those who were suffering from nocturnal starvation because his aphrodisiacs had failed to work on their husbands.

When Mrs. Giscobbe had gone, the doctor asked Petrillo if he liked the look of her, and when the tailor said, "Sure," the doctor answered, "Good, because I've got a plan which will cure our corner of the Depression for us.

"You start something going with Mrs. G. Later, I'll give her something fatal to put in her husband's drink."

"But that's murder."

"That's the only way we'll get the insurance."

"I like it."

Petrillo wooed and won Mrs. Giscobbe, an easy accomplishment, and while they were stoking the fires of love, the doctor was quoting the fires of hate to Mrs. Giscobbe, by letting her know what Tony was up to elsewhere. Meanwhile, Petrillo was telling his new love how nice it would be if Tony wasn't around because then they could be together all the time. Mrs. Giscobbe was also apprised of the fact that if Tony even left to live with the girl who had become his exclusive mistress, she would lose the store and the insurance. Dr. Bolber chose hemlock to put Tony down, on the theory that what was good enough for a great philosopher, was good enough for an illiterate grocer.

Hemlock – or conium – kills by greatly exaggerating any illness the victim may already have, so the first thing to do was to give Tony an ailment. He was in the habit of coming home in the early hours, more or less incapable with drink. So incapable, in fact, that he could hardly get into bed properly. The lovers waited until the right night; until Tony was really loaded. Then they undressed him and left him naked on the bed with the window wide open. It was a bad winter that year and in the morning Tony woke up with something approaching pneumonia.

A doctor, but not Bolber, was called, and left medicines. Mrs. Giscobbe carried these to Dr. Bolber's office and waited while he spiked them with hemlock. When Tony died, the family doctor had to admit that he wasn't surprised. "Your husband was an alcoholic, Mrs. Giscobbe, and they often succumb to pneumonia."

The insurance company paid out $10,000 without a moment's hesitation, and Mrs. Giscobbe gave half to the doctor. In a few days, however, she was again back in the surgery, in tears, saying that the tailor no longer fancied her. Dr. Bolber was ready with a line of patter. He was keeping Petrillo in reserve for other things. He told the widow that she had $5,000, a fine grocery store and a prospect more worthy than her fickle tailor would presently present himself. This is what eventually happened. Mrs. Giscobbe wouldn't be heard of again until the doctor's arrest, but that was many years away. He showed her to the door, telling her to drop in when the new man in her life arrived, so that he could give her a little something to make cupid bite, so to speak, but she never came back.

Dr. Bolber, a man of vision, realised that he was on to a good thing. What with the handsome Petrillo and the fast-killing hemlock, a new business had opened up before him. He even envisaged the day when he could have branch offices in every major city.

Paul Petrillo next took up with a Maria Lorenzo, the wife of a building worker. So attentive was the tailor that Maria was soon complaining about what a terrible bore her husband was. In the meantime, the doctor was having trouble finding clients, not so much because they didn't want to play the game, but because there was no insurance money in the background for him to gain as prize money. The doctor was made aware of the simple, brutal truth that the poor Italians simply couldn't afford insurance.

Petrillo had the next bright idea. "Why don't we insure some of them? We can begin with Maria's husband."

But Bolber saw the problem. You just couldn't insure somebody without them knowing. There had to be a medical and the prospect had to sign the papers.

Petrillo said, "What we need is a good actor."

Bolber clicked his fingers. "That's it. What about your cousin Herman?"

Before he had gone into counterfeiting, Herman Petrillo, (as he was always reminding people), had been an actor. When he heard about the caper, he was quite willing to play the part of a construction worker named Lorenzo.

Dr. Bolber had another idea – given to him by Lorenzo's profession. Accidental death brought a double insurance, so he decided, when the moment came, that Lorenzo would be pushed off one of the roofs which he was repairing.

When Paul Petrillo had pushed his affair with Maria to a fine pitch, and she was confessing that if only Lorenzo was gone she would marry him, he told her that her husband's disappearance could be arranged. But it would be a pity, after all the sacrifices and indignities she had faced in the marriage, that Lorenzo couldn't leave her a nest-egg with which to start her new life.

A plan was hatched, and while Lorenzo was repairing a roof in another part of the city, the actor, Petrillo, got up to look like him in a dishevelled shirt and down-at-heel carpet slippers was seeing a Prudential Insurance Company official at Maria's home. Herman signed for the insurance, paid the first quarter's instalment, and was in the Lorenzo home a few days later for the insurance company doctor to give him a medical check-up.

Meanwhile, Herman also made it his business to drink where Lorenzo drank, and they became fast friends. Lorenzo liked looking at pornographic pictures, which was a coincidence, Herman said, because so did he, and he had plenty. Bolber didn't give the word to Herman to kill his new friend until a second instalment had been paid on the insurance policy. Then "Happy" Herman climbed to the roof where Lorenzo was working. He had just got some terrific art work, he said, so he had rushed up to show Lorenzo. Lorenzo looked down at the photographs, but then kept going straight down, for all eight floors, as Herman gave him a hefty shove.

It was six months before Herman called on Bolber again. The doctor, who had a notorious reputation for taciturnity, said, "Can you swim?"

"Sure thing."

"Good. You're going fishing."

Herman read a couple of fishing books and bought some tackle. His mark was an Italian named Fierenza. Not only was he a man who fished as a hobby but his wife just happened to be Paul's latest mistress. There was $5,000 insurance on Fierenza, with a double indemnity if he died in an accident. A new face showed up on the next few Sundays among the crowd who fished at the Schuylkill River. Mr. Fierenza particularly noticed Herman because he was so friendly and always gave him – and the others – a friendly nod.

One day, which happened to be Fierenza's last, he was just about to get into a boat when the friendly man came up. "You going out alone?"

"Yes."

"Whyn't let me share it with you? We can split the cost." "Also," here he slapped his hip, "I have a bottle." Herman knew that Fierenza was partial to a drink. He had also been told that he couldn't swim.

They anchored in a secluded corner of the river. Herman was cautious. It might be that the doctor had got the facts wrong. Better safe than sorry.

"Can you swim?" Herman asked.

Shame-faced, Fierenza admitted that he couldn't.

Herman suddenly pointed to something behind his companion. "Hey!" he said, with just the right note of alarm, "What's that?" Fierenza turned to look – and Herman lifted him and threw him over the side.

Herman followed him in, so that being wet, it would look as though he had attempted a rescue. Actually, he swung under the boat, grabbed Fierenza's kicking legs and dragged him down.

Later, distraught and soaked, Herman arrived back on shore and, the perfect actor still, gabbled an incoherent story of how his companion had died. "I think his name was Fierenza," Herman told the police. "I don't really know. I hardly knew the guy."

The police didn't suspect murder because the men were almost strangers. What would have been the motive? And Paul Petrillo used this as an excuse to ease himself out of any permanent relationship with the widow. "We wouldn't want the cops to know that the man who was with your husband when he died was your lover's cousin."

The ambitious Dr. Bolber was all for expansion. Things weren't progressing as fast as he would have liked. It happened that there lived in another corner of Philadelphia, a witch of a woman named Carino Favato. She was in much the same line of business as Bolber. Known affectionately as *The Witch*, she supplied the superstitious and illiterate Italians in North Philadelphia with love potions, saltpeter and aphrodisiacs. Lurid rumour had it, although these things are rarely checked out, that this obese, hook-nosed creature had buried three of her five husbands after poisoning them.

Dr. Bolber popped round for a social visit one Sunday and the talk eventually turned to business. The only difference between them seemed to be that *The Witch* preferred arsenic as a spouse-remover. "What about the double indemnity, though?" prompted Bolber.

She hadn't thought about that. Bolber also boasted that he didn't wait for the initiative to come from neglected wives, but went straight to them. He asked the old woman if she knew of any wives whose relationship with their husbands was weak, and who had a corresponding weakness in the head, heart and morality department. Eager for a share in the profits, Carino Favato came up with a Mrs. Petrino whose husband, Dominic, a janitor, was spending more time in the bedrooms of the tenants than of his wife. Paul Petrillo was now sent for and got to work on the neglected wife almost immediately. Herman arrived next and was posing as Dominic, in shirt sleeves and slippers, when the "Man from the Pru" called. There was one problem. The salesman wanted to know how a janitor, not one of the best paying of jobs, could afford such hefty insurance. Bolber had sent Herman to the interview with false bank books which showed the Petrinos were worth twelve thousand dollars. Herman said they dabbled successfully in real estate.

There was a slight shock, however, when (a little later) he was checked out by the company's doctor. "I seem to know you?" said the doctor. It was the same medical man who had examined him on the other side of the city, when he had taken out a policy in the name of Lorenzo.

Herman, as accomplished as a wit as he was an actor, replied, "I don't think so. But you know what they say – all us Italians look alike."

An instalment or so later, Dr. Bolber gave Herman the nod. Herman waited for Dominic at the top of a flight of metal steps. It was dark and Herman was gripping a huge spanner. Once

Dominic had come up the stairs, he soon went down again. It was decided that the janitor had slipped in the dark and fractured his skull.

The Witch took her $500 with one hand and slipped Dr. Bolber a piece of paper with the name of a new prospect written on it with the other. This was a street fish peddler named Luigi Primavera. Again the Petrillos moved into action; more smoothly now because they were experienced. Paul seduced the wife while Herman posed as the fishmonger. The only difference was in the last reel of the drama. Dr. Bolber felt like an officer stuck behind the lines at headquarters. He wanted to see a little action so he decided to put down the fishmonger himself. It had to be an accidental death as he was still going for a double pay out.

A dark night found Dr. Bolber waiting behind the wheel of a car, complete with fake licence plates, in the southern section of the city. It was raining and the streets were deserted. Eventually he saw Luigi Primavera, back bent, pushing his heavy handcart along the street. Dr. Bolber followed him for a time and waited while he made house deliveries.

Bolber saw his chance when the fishmonger was trudging back across the street. He gunned the engine, the car roared forward over the rainsoaked, glistening roadway, and Bolber felt like a Hollywood gangster as the automobile rocketed along the road. But Luigi moved faster in the street than he apparently did in bed, and managed to get right up on the pavement before Bolber reached him. He had probably half swung round, seen the doctor, and realised that it was a deliberate attempt on his life. There was nothing for Bolber to do but reverse a little, chase the fishmonger up on the sidwalk and hammer him against the railings.

A few witnesses saw the incident. Luigi couldn't talk about it. He was dead. But all papers carried stories of the hit-and-run killer and voiced the suspicion that it might not have been only an unfortunate accident.

Dr. Bolber spent an anxious few days pacing his office and swearing that if only cops didn't come for him, he would never do a criminal act again. He was in luck. Neither the police, nor the insurance investigators, were suspicious, and Mrs. Primavera picked up her double indemnity.

It was said that the doctor felt so badly living this dire crisis that he went to another doctor for a check-up and was warned that he was overworking. But Dr. Bolber had had a shock and he decided to moderate his actions. The number of victims, of course, wouldn't be reduced. They would still handle every project they could find, but in future they wouldn't go for the risky double indemnity which needed an accidental death. Instead, future victims would be foully destroyed in a manner which suggested *natural death*. And, Dr. Bolber told his confederates at a conference, he had been experimenting, and had discovered just the way to do it. It involved the use of a canvas sack containing twenty pounds of sand. One blow from this sack, said the doctor, would render a victim unconscious; and any repeated blows would bring about death by cerebral haemorrhage. The beauty of it was that no traces would show. There would be hardly any bruising, if any, on the skull. The confederates were delighted. They thought the doctor's invention a knockout and, it was said, Happy Herman, peeved because the doctor had handled the Primavera business, was anxious to be the first to try it.

Nemesis didn't come to the gang for another five years and during that time, it was estimated that they killed some thirty people. Their victims were usually poor Italians, the new immigrants who lived in the city's teeming slums, and nobody paid any interest when they died; even when their deaths were tinged with suspicion. The Italians, most of whom could speak only a few words of English, didn't feel confident enough to carry any doubts that they might have had to the authorities, and in those days there were no social workers to look after and listen to the complaints of these people.

The doctor and the Petrillos were living in some style. Even *The Witch* was splashing money about in the only way she knew how; she had never missed a baseball match but now she always had a box to herself, and during the game wolfed down hot-dogs by the dozen.

It was a tip-off from an ex-prisoner which led to the ultimate investigation and exposure of the murderers. In the spring of 1937 a convict named Harrison was finishing his sentence. During his incarceration he had invented a new cleansing liquid, and his companions had told him to see Herman Petrillo on his release as he had both money and influence and might back the fluid's production and marketing.

Harrison went to see Petrillo. Herman decided to take the released con on a magnificent drunk because he himself had once done time and knew exactly how a man felt on his release. But Herman drank too much and became indiscreet. He told Harrison he wasn't interested in financing cleaning fluid, it was too speculative, and besides which, it was legitimate. But he told Harrison that he found him an agreeable person and would like to put some business his way. "Look, I'll tell you what to do. You go find a lonely guy who has no friends or relatives and on whom we can take out some insurance. After that, we'll knock him off, and you'll get a share of the money."

Harrison went to the police. There had been whispers before, of course, about a murder-for-insurance group working in the city, but the slums threw up many of these lurid rumours. The first man the police watched was Herman. Herman didn't seem to have any work but he always had plenty of money. Eventually they arrested him on suspicion of murder, and got the newspapers to publicise the arrest. One of the first people to recognise Herman's photograph in the press, was the insurance doctor who had twice medically examined him under the names of Lorenzo and Petrino.

The next steps were logical, and the widows Lorenzo and Petrino were arrested. They were soon talking, and principally about handsome Paul Petrillo, Herman's cousin. Soon the Petrillo cousins were each trying to out-sing the other in order to save their lives; throwing up names and dates like a couple of computers. There were soon convoys of not so merry widows arriving under a police escort.

Strangely enough, the murders didn't attract great attention. These were just the money-grabbing goings-on-among-rapacious-immigrants, newspaper editors seem to have decided. They had no real news value because after all, it was the sort of thing one could expect.

Dr. Bolber and *The Witch* were arrested. Nobody made things difficult for the police by refusing to talk. The Petrillo cousins came off worst. They were sentenced to death and eventually executed. The doctor and the old woman were luckier. They only got life.

DR. MARCEL PETIOT

Nobody will ever be sure how many dozens of people the French doctor Marcel Petiot poisoned. Certainly among the doctors in this book he is the highest scorer, the ace of aces. At his trial in Paris in 1946, he was found guilty of murdering twenty-four, and he confessed that he thought the figure, give or take one or two, was sixty-three. But when he made this admission, he was hoping posterity wouldn't look on him too unkindly, and it is probably that the death toll was around the hundred mark. Moreover, since he was held prisoner by the Gestapo for a time, Petiot ran up his high score in some fifteen short months. The fact that the times were unusual and conditions chaotic – because Paris was occupied by the German Army – doesn't really detract from Petiot's outrageous audacity. It just shows, supreme opportunist that he was, that he exploited every possible advantage.

With the cocky confidence of the drug addict, Marcel Petiot tried to pose as a hero to the Gestapo by claiming he was destroying Jews and Communists. But when captured by the French he maintained that all the people he had put down with poison were German soldiers or French traitors collaborating with the enemy. Having failed to get the German Iron Cross, he tried for the French Croix de Geurre and a hero's welcome instead of Madame Guillotine. If the facts that follow sound exaggerated, let me assure you that they are true in all salient points and clearly prove that old adage that truth is often stranger than fiction.

Much about Petiot still remains unknown. Some of this is because of the wartime conditions that prevailed when he was carrying out his crimes, and the fact that what the Gestapo said or did in connection with the dapper doctor, nobody probably lived to tell. Another factor seems to be that the French, unlike the English, the Americans and the Germans seem not to revere their famous murderers, and no reporter has considered it worthwhile to back-track over Petiot's extraordinary life.

If France can be said to be, traditionally, the home of Bluebeards, Dr. Petriot can be said to be their king. Yet his criminal activities for most of his career were mundane enough, and were made the less notorious because of his undoubted gifts as a medical man, and because of his many acts of kindness to the unfortunate. Petiot was a petty thief, he was also a sexual pervert. But so clever was Petiot – and so kind – that his neighbours mostly made allowances for the bad side of his character and put it down to a brilliant man's eccentricities.

But this, of course, was long before Paris and the abnormal conditions caused by the German Occupation that permitted the doctor to murder on a mass scale. Had these conditions not existed it is probable that we would never have heard of Dr. Petiot. He would have murdered perhaps five or six people in the course of a busy life in his profession. Never to have been found out, he would have died in obscurity, forgotten by all but his loved ones. For Petiot, unlike many compulsive murderers, valued his skin, and could contain his sadism and his lust for profit if there seemed to be any risk involved. Cunning kept Petiot alive and enabled him to kill close to a hundred unfortunates who had turned to him for help while fleeing from the Gestapo. It was cunning that kept the dapper doctor with the bushy hair, the over-white facial skin, the pushy and pompous manner, and with an eloquence of speech, popular, respected and trusted while the list of his victims spiralled upwards.

Marcel Petiot was born in 1897 in Auxerre, a village some hundred miles south of Paris. He was the son of a minor postal official. He showed a brilliance at school which enabled him to glide through his examinations, while at the same time having a penchant for petty larceny against his school chums. A juvenile sadism had him carrying out experiments on animals and insects. In his teens he was committing acts of burglary around the village and showing, some thought, an unnatural interest in the human body and the methods with which to torment and repair it. Petiot himself, however, excused this fascination on the grounds that it was his ambition to become a doctor and therefore he must know all about these things.

In 1917 Petiot was conscripted into the Army, and was wounded in the Argonne. It has also been said that at about this time he was stealing morphine from a casualty clearing station and peddling it to addicts in the Dijon area. The Army obviously found something wrong with him, for they discharged him with a pension and instructions to undergo psychoneurosis treatment. He spent the next two years either in an asylum or loafing about at home. Yet he still managed to study medicine and even to qualify early in 1921.

His mother was baffled by his brilliance and his speed in digesting medical subjects. She had seen him do nothing in the year he was supposed to be studying, but drift aimlessly about the house and sleep.

Dr. Petiot took a practice at the small town of Villeneuve Sur Yonne, which was twenty-five miles from his home. It had a population of some 5,000 people, and Petiot soon became a hero to the poor and a villian to the rich. If a sufferer couldn't afford the treatment, Petiot would tell him to pay for it if and when he could; in the meantime, he would charge his better off patients extra.

At about this time, however, while still in his twenties, it is possible that Petiot might have chalked up his first murder. The victim was a pretty girl who came to him as his housekeeper. It was being noted some months later that she looked ripely pregnant.

Neighbours were most specific that not only *was* the maid pregnant but that in addition she was seen crying a lot. A Madame Fleury told the police that she had heard Petiot threatening the girl with violence if she didn't blame her condition on the town idiot, a man who was mostly drunk and insensible. The doctor promptly answered Madame Fleury's charge by saying she had been romantically interested in him (he had declined the offer) and that she was acting as a woman scorned. The police seemed to have believed the mayor. The maid vanished and the gossips found other topics.

Other women visited Petiot, and soon the neighbours were again exchanging spicy gossip to the effect that women could be heard crying in torment through the doctor's open windows. The word got around that Petiot went in for sadistic practices. But if this was so, the visitors never complained, indeed, they were often seen calling again. And after all, Petiot was popular. In fact he was so popular, despite the many stories told about him, that he stood as a candidate for the local government, and was elected the mayor of the town.

At this time (1928) he already had a lurid reputation in the town, if the gossip after his arrest and exposure is to be believed. But if village history, unrecorded at the time, grows with retelling down the long years, the stories are no less fantastic than what we know about his crimes. Thus, there are reports of a second murder. A mother who complained because Petiot had encouraged her daughter's drug addiction died suddenly and mysteriously. Around this time he married Georgette, the pretty daughter of a Parisien restauranteur.

Meanwhile, it is said, the mayor continued his habits of petty

larceny about the town as well as indulging in a little Peeping
Tommery. If he was ever caught peering into a window at a
nocturnal hour, he could always say, I suppose, that he was
indulging in a bit of long-range patient study. The gossip about
him continued and some of it stuck. In 1930, for example, a
Madame Debauve was found murdered and robbed. Rumour
said Petiot was the villain. A woman who was loud in the cam-
paign against the doctor was also being treated by him for rheumatism. All talk stopped when she died suddenly, and perhaps
reluctantly, the gossips turned once more to other subjects.
Petiot had by this time certainly become a colourfully eccentric
figure, with vehement supporters as well as detractors, and a
discussion about him at the cafe's was certain to brighten the
duller hours.

In 1930 there was another sensation, this time factually sup-
ported, when Petiot was arrested for both burglarising his own
electric meter and stealing, in his capacity as mayor, from the
municipal store. He went to prison for a short time, and to escape
the shame, Georgette scurried for the anonymity of Paris with
their son.

On his release, Petiot started a practice in the Opera district
of Paris, at 66 Rue Caumartin. From the start, to the horror of
the other doctors in the district, he was a blazing success. The
reasons for this were two-fold. He was undoubtedly a gifted
doctor who could even diagnose accurately and swiftly in
instances where other physicians had reported themselves
mystified. That was the credit side of his record. The second
reason for his success, the debit side (which made him rich) was
that he busied himself ending unwanted pregnancies and supply-
ing drugs to addicts.

He was in trouble with the police once more when he stole a
book from a bookshop, but was let off providing he underwent
psychiatric treatment. Petiot said he would take care of the medical side of Petiot himself. He never trusted doctors, he said,
because he knew too much about them. It is safe to assume, like
so many other doctors in this book, that Petiot, already a
shaky personality, was undermining what little sanity he had
left by a daily dosage of a dangerous drug.

But in the summer of 1939, when the war clouds gathered,
Dr. Petiot was both popular and prosperous. It was said he had
accounts in twenty banks. He was admired by his neighbours;
was seen in church each Sunday with Georgette and his son,
and was even known to read the Bible in his surgery while he
waited for the next patient.

Then the war came. Paris became a city of unrest and conflict.

Armed fascists, who were against the war, terrorised the city for a time. Things quietened down through the "Phoney War" period, and then the German Army struck through Belgium and invaded France. Hermann Goring's Stukas blasted a way for von Rundstedt's tanks and within weeks Dr. Petiot could hear the measured tread of marching jackboots from his surgery window.

France had fallen, Paris was occupied. It is hard to imagine the effect this must have had on the citizens of Paris, and on Dr. Petiot in particular. One wonders if this was a key factor in completely shattering what was left of his drug-battered sanity.

The occupation, of course, was like no other known in Europe in modern times. The ordinary German troops were well behaved, but with them they brought a new kind of animal, a political, racist thug, in a Gestapo uniform, who was everywhere: watching, waiting, seizing, torturing and killing.

Dr. Petiot's surgery continued. If anything he had more work to do as strain brought more patients to him with complaints. Women sought the termination of their pregnancies rather than have children in a world that seemed to have gone mad. And it was now that Dr. Petiot, so deceptively sane on the surface, began to commit murder on a mass scale. His first victim, ironically, was the man who gave him the germ which became the idea. He was a Pole, a Jewish refugee named Joachim Gusbinov, a neighbour on the Rue Caumartin. It might be that Petiot had been boasting about imaginary connections he had with the French Resistance Movement, or it might have been that Gusbinov, sensing the fate which awaited all Jews in occupied Europe, broached the matter first.

He asked Petiot if he knew any way he could get himself smuggled out of Europe to South America. Petiot suggested there might be a way but it could be prohibitively expensive. Gusbinov said any expense was worth it, and Petiot told the Pole to leave the matter with him and he would make inquiries. These inquiries began and stopped with Petiot and the underground escape route began and ended in a house that the doctor purchased in the Etoile district of Paris at 21 Rue Lesueur.

The building was a villa, and had once been the property of a Russian princess. It had a garden and a large garage, as well as its own furnace for creating heat and hot water. Petiot contracted local builders to carry out alterations. He told them he was taking over the property to convert it into a private hospital for mentally retarded patients. But even so the builders must have wondered why he needed some of the alterations demanded.

There were two small rooms at the rear of the garage. One of these was a peculiarly triangular shape. It was also windowless. Petiot had a spyhole made in the door and a false door fitted on the opposite wall. A large pit was dug in the garage floor and covered with boards and a trapdoor. Petiot also wanted a more powerful furnace to supply water and heat to his patients and the builders suggested another furnace be installed. A garden wall was heightened so that neighbours couldn't see into the grounds.

By January 1942, some three months after Gusbinov first raised the matter, Dr. Petiot was ready to go into the liquidating business for the double purpose of profit and perverted sexual pleasure. He told the Pole that he had made contacts with the Resistance Movement, there was an escape route, but it would cost two million francs – not for the Resistance, of course – but to bribe border guards, officials and seamen, and to pay for his passage to South America.

Gusbinov eagerly agreed to the terms and Petiot told him to go to the Rue Lesueur address late at night, taking his money and whatever other possessions he needed with him. Petiot was there to meet him. He took his friend to the garage, to await the agents with the transportation, and then Patriot remembered something: "I ought to give you an injection against smallpox, Joachim, so there won't be any problems when you arrive in South America."

Gusbinov must have thanked Petiot for thinking of the matter at such a fraught moment, and he promptly rolled up his sleeve. After giving him the injection, Petiot would have told him to lay down and rest in the small room, and locking the door, Petiot would have taken up his position at the spyhole to watch the death agony. After calling in vain for help, the Pole, in great agony, would have tried the doors – the one where Petiot watched and the false one, and failing in these he would have torn his fingers in trying to claw his way through the roughcast brick. It was a macabre play that Petiot would watch, tirelessly and without mercy, some sixty-three times. Not only single men would go into the small room to rest but at times entire families, including women and children. The fleeing Jews not only had Adolf Eichman, with his efficient railway to the liquidation camps to contend with, they had Dr. Petiot, and he arrived on the scene when they thought they had reached a measure of safety and had the protection of a friend.

When his victims were dead, Petiot briskly and efficiently removed them to the furnace. He kept all their possessions neatly stacking their clothing in racks, according to sizes and sexes. He would leave the bodies burning in the furnace and drive back on his motorcycle to his Caumartin surgery. A day or so later, he would return to the furnace and remove what was left to the pit in the cellar, which had been topped up with lime. The need for a plentiful supply of quicklime was to be a perpetual headache for him, and was bound to make people curious.

Madame Gusbinov received a visit from Petiot a day after her husband had started on his journey. The doctor told her Joachim had gone and gave her the torn half a a hundred franc note. "When I give you the second half, madame, you will know your husband is safely in South America." It was a piece of bizarre theatre he would use with all the nearest and dearest of his victims. Madame Gusbinov, looking back several years later, recalled how she had thanked the doctor for his kindness and how, gruff with embarrassment, Petiot claimed (the epitome of modesty for once) that he had only done his duty.

There were more known victims in swift succession. One was a pimp named Jean Marc Van Bever who was a drug addict. He came to Petiot for supplies but couldn't pay because his girl was in prison. Petiot refused him the drug. The pimp threatened to go to the authorities and tell them he was a peddler. Petiot relented and said, "All right, but you'll have to go to my other surgery. I now keep the dangerous stuff there." A few weeks later the prostitute asked Petiot if he had seen her man. "Yes," Petiot answered laconically, "The Gestapo have got him."

Nobody ever bothered to ask what had happened to the pimp after that. People disappeared after seeing the Gestapo – and nobody dared inquire.

Another early victim was known to be Dr. Paul Braunberger, a wealthy refugee who also practised medicine on the Rue Caumartin. The murder might have been purely for profit, it might have been that Petiot wanted the refugee's practice, or it might be that he had tired of his doctor friend and of playing cards with him several nights a week. It could well have been a combination of all three motives which made Petiot decide that Dr. Paul Braunberger had to go.

Dr. Braunberger wouldn't have needed much convincing. He was uneasy about the German presence in France along with the thousands of other refugees sheltering in the country. Although at this point in time, the Spring of 1942, the Germans had not yet made any overt threat against the refugees, commonsense would have told them it was just a matter of time and organisation before they did. There would have been no street-level knowledge about Hitler's secret directive for the liquidation of the European Jews, but the mood was there to be sensed. In all the other places the Jews were being harassed or taken into captivity, and Dr. Braunberger knew that the Germans were only needing a little more confidence before they turned on the Jews in Paris.

Petiot met no hesitation therefore when, during a card game with Braunberger, he said, "I think it would be healthier for you, old friend, if you fled France." Braunberger agreed, but the question was how. Petiot added: "There are ways and means. It will cost two million francs – that's not for me or the Resistance, you understand, but for those people on the escape route who are motivated by greed not humanity."

Dr. Braunberger eagerly agreed to leave the details to Petiot and one night he was summoned to the house in Rue Leseur along with his two million francs and his other possessions. Two years later his favourite pack of cards would be identified amongst the stack of possessions found there.

Next, it is known, an entire family, the Knellers, went through Petiot's escape route and the doctor became enriched by £15,000 in the process.

There was only one thing causing Petiot concern at this time. The deliveries of quicklime. The local dealer from whom he ordered supplies was curious, especially as Petiot always demanded that the loads be delivered at night. Petiot told the man he needed the lime for experiments, then decided to cancel future orders by saying his experiments had finished. Petiot next arranged that his brother Maurice, who lived in Auxerre, should bring him supplies. A sudden call would come in the night. "Bring a load of quicklime, quickly, Maurice," Petiot would say.

Eventually, when Petiot was a prisoner of the Gestapo, Maurice Petiot would visit Paris and pay a visit to the private hospital. He didn't stay long and when he returned to Auxerre he had nothing to say but, it is said, he looked a shaken man, a changed man. People put it down, like they put most changes down, to the damned war.

The neighbours in the quiet street often saw Dr. Petiot noisily racing to and from his private hospital. If they never saw any patients arrive in the day or heard them playing in the grounds, they too probably blamed the war. The doctor wouldn't open up perhaps, until the Germans had gone. Soon, Petiot was employing touts to tour the boulevard cafes to find him refugees who wished to flee the country and could pay for the privilege. The touts, of course, didn't know what really happened. They thought Petiot was in the business for either patriotism or profit or a bit of both. When the next-of-kin stayed behind Petiot never forgot his melodramatic little touch of delivering a torn half of a 100-franc note, and reminding them that when he presented them with the second half they would know their loved one was safe. He went right through nearly a hundred victims using this method, never once giving away the wrong half of the note.

One can visualise the monster, as efficient in his office as an Adolf Eichmann, carefully tucking half a note in an envelope and putting it to one side with the victim's name on it so there wouldn't be any slip-ups. And visualise him, not too tidily it would transpire, seeing that there was lumber in plenty for the furnaces, quicklime for the pit (which he told Maurice he needed to whitewash the walls Paris being such a grimy city) and sweeping out the triangle room for the next temporary incumbent.

Petiot had something like a sixteen-month uninterrupted run of success in which he must have been disposing of refugees at the rate of two or three a week. Then a peculiar irony happened. The Gestapo came for him, rushed him to a deep cell and put him through a fierce interrogation. The Gestapo had heard rumours that Petiot was running an escape channel for refugees and other wanted criminals. They had even tested it, they said. The Gestapo had bribed a Jew to approach Petiot for help in escaping. Now the Jew had disappeared and the only conclusion the Gestapo could reach was that Petiot had got the man away.

Petiot was faced with a dilemma. What would happen if he told them the truth? More to the point, he would know what would happen if he didn't. If he confessed, you never knew with Nazis. They might turn him over to the French authorities for mass murder, a trial and the guillotine. But if he remained silent it was certain torture and bullets from a German firing squad would follow. The feeling in Paris is that Petiot told the Gestapo the truth, told them he was on their side, doing his modest little bit to solve the Jewish Question, by ridding the world of rich refugees.

All the signs indicate, as fantastic as it may sound, that Petiot did indeed tell them the truth. It was true he remained in prison for some six or seven months, but he must have given the Germans a problem. No doubt they checked and there was evidence in plenty at the private hospital. But not only didn't they shoot him or turn him over to the French authorities, they eventually released him and it was unlike the Gestapo to release anybody who they had evidence against.

The assumption can only be that he confessed and the Germans, after recovering from their astonishment and amusement, and checking with Berlin, had released him. Berlin faced a quandary. Petiot was undoubtedly a lunatic, a killer for profit and pleasure, but in Nazi philosophy he was committing no crime because his victims were people fleeing the Germans for one reason or another.

Dr. Petiot was an asset, whatever his motives, for he was destroying their enemies for them.

Moreover the higher echelon of the Gestapo knew something that Petiot didn't know, something which would have made him confident. The efficient Adolf Eichmann, with a set of elaborate railway time-tables, was arranging for the shipment of all Jews to extermination camps in Poland and Germany. One wonders if Eichmann was informed of the mad doctor's modest efforts in the same direction, and one can imagine him chuckling over the story while ordering Petiot's immediate release so he could return to the good work.

But what we do know is that the Gestapo held Petiot for some seven months while the issue was secretly debated, and then they sent him back, without any curb on his movements, to business. It seemed to be a green light for Petiot. He couldn't wait to get the furnaces stoked up again. He was arrested in May 1943 and he was released by the Germans in the Christmas period of the same year. In February 1944, we know, Petiot hurriedly contacted his brother Maurice by telephone because he needed a delivery of quicklime, urgently. His brother, without telling Marcel the ghastly things he had seen on his visit to the private hospital, apparently refused to help. Petiot decided to do without the quicklime, which indicated the confidence he now felt. Could it be that with the support of the German conquerors, he now thought it didn't matter too much if the truth came out? After all, the Germans had the power to protect him from his own, defeated people.

Petiot must have given a Gallic shrug, dismissed the matter and busied himself about the hospital. Apparently, in his months of absence, his touts had been energetic and there was a queue of refugees waiting to escape. But his over-confidence, we assume given him by his German captors, led to his undoing. His production was too much for his facilities, which had worried the arch-exterminator Eichmann in his early days. Petiot's chimneys began to smoke in the day as well as at night, jettisoning columns of black greasy smoke incessantly into the early sunshine. Old soldiers in the neighbourhood sniffed a sweetish spring smell lingering in the air, a sick sweetish smell which reminded them of abandoned trenches on hotly-contested battlefields.

The smell was, unmistakably, of decaying flesh, and neighbours complained, and *le exterminator petit* made some attempt to solve the problem by only stocking up the fires at night. On a miniscule scale, he had Colonel Eichmann's problem but Eichmann had all the industrial resources of Germany behind him, Petiot was a one-man private enterprise. And the touts, working energetically, were finding more refugees and, with the mean soul of the peasant, or just because of pride, Petiot hated to turn anybody away.

He couldn't improve on his facilities and he was still working without quicklime. The complaints forgotten, Petiot's chimneys were soon billowing greasy black smoke again.

Petiot was working too hard by now. Georgette, his trusting wife, was the first to notice it and urge him to slow down. He was attempting too much, she said, running two surgeries and working dangerously with the Underground. Georgette, when the truth became known, would refuse to believe it, stoutly maintaining that if anybody was killed by her husband it was for the glory of France. Petiot certainly looked tired during his last few weeks of freedom. He was rushing hither and wither on his little red motorcycle, and friends and neighbours, misunderstanding the reasons now the Second Front was expected, made clucking noises of sympathy.

When Petiot was away all evening and not returning until the early hours, then only to collapse, a spent force on the bed, falling asleep as soon as his head hit pillow, Georgette gained comfort from the fact that the francs were piling up at an amazing rate in the bank. "At least I know he loves me still," she would tell her friends, "and it's not another woman who keeps him from me."

Petiot's lack of professional resources caused the trouble. He was one brain, two furnaces, one pit, and his touts were too efficient. A shadow of his former self, his weight having shrunk, Petiot stoked up his two furnaces to a fearsome blaze on Saturday. March 11, 1944, and mounting his red motorcycle raced through the night for his Rue Caumartin surgery to attend to his patients there.

He had neglected to have the chimneys swept and they caught alight. Soon the neighbourhood was wreathed in black smoke as thick as porridge. A neighbour, M. Jaques Marcais, reached for the phone and complained angrily to the police. A sergeant arrived, called in several other gendarmes and spoke to the neighbours who had now gathered in the street. There was a note pinned on the door of the private hospital which directed any inquiries to Dr. Petiot at his Rue Caumartin surgery.

The sergeant phoned Petiot, told him the problem and Petiot breezily said he would come over to attend to it. But Petiot seemed to have delayed. The blaze became worse and the sergeant called in the fire brigade.

When the little exterminator finally did charge up on his

motorcycle the police and the firemen were already in the cellar. While the firemen were hosing the flames, the police sergeant was trying to calculate how many bits and pieces of body, skull and limbs there were in the cellar and how many people, if they were reassembled, they would make up to be.

Petiot, seeing the situation, didn't turn and run for it. Petiot had never been short with an answer in his life and he wasn't about to start now. Calmly he led the sergeant to one side, away from the other listeners, and gave his explanation. "You must understand, sergeant," he said, "this is war and somebody has to do the unpleasant work. Since I am a doctor I had to do my duty and volunteer for the job."

His explanation, he was the disposal unit for the French Resistance Movement. These human remains had been German soldiers, he said, and French traitors who had been condemned to death for collaborating with the enemies of France. "If I deserve anything at all" he declared, "it is a medal, not a prison cell." He added that it hadn't been easy to carry out such gruesome work, even on traitors, and the sergeant had that evidence before him in Petiot's bloodshot eyes, emaciated appearance and over-white skin.

Petiot was permitted to go but the sergeant said he must, of course, report the matter to his superiors.

"You must be discreet, sergeant," Petiot declared.

The officer said he would be discreet, Petiot had nothing to fear, for the Gestapo would never hear of the matter. But, naturally, it must be reported.

Petiot seemed satisfied with this, mounted his motorcycle and roared away. The sergeant relayed his story. No doubt his superiors made a few discreet telephone calls and found out that the French Resistance Movement didn't have a Monsieur Petiot, and if there had been any liquidation of traitors they would hardly be in such numbers, nor would they be executed at one place.

In the middle of the night, carloads of detectives arrived outside the private hospital. They found enough clothes in cupboards to open a secondhand clothes shop. They found enough pieces of jewellery and other personal possessions to bankrupt a pawn-broker. What surprised them was the childrens clothes. Children sentenced to death for collaborating with the enemy? That was a good one. The doctor had kept copious notes of his victims. There were lists of names and dates and these the police assumed to be the people who had died in the cellar. They found the pit and the remains of dozens of bodies. In the cellar, awaiting a turn in the furnaces, were an estimated twenty-four bodies (Petiot would say it was twenty-seven), all of whom had been cut up into manageable chunks like logs of wood.

The detectives were intrigued by the names on the lists, for most of them seemed of Jewish and Polish and German extraction. Jews collaborating with the Germans? That was another funny one. The police decided that Petiot was an exterminator working for the Germans, and, despite what the Gestapo might say, they went through the motions of arresting and holding him for mass murder.

But before they could arrest him they had to find him. Petiot had hurried home, told Georgette to pack and left for Auxerre with his wife and grown-up son. He spent just one night with Maurice, his curious brother, and then leaving Georgette and his son there, disappeared. His story was that the Gestapo were after him again. His next stop was Paris, following the sound criminal principle that the best place to disappear was in a large city.

He hid in the house of a friend, a housepainter named Georges Redoute, on the Rue Faubourg St Denis, in a suburb on the outskirts of Paris. But it wasn't like Petiot to self-efface himself even when he was in hiding. He soon became a notorious nuisance in the area because of his habit of standing bare-chested at the open window. The locals nick-named him Tarzan.

Police were hampered by the fact that his dossier had disappeared back at the village of Villeneuve, where he had been mayor until 1930. The Gestapo, having heard that Petiot was hunted and believed to be their Paris exterminator, denied all knowledge of him and encouraged the French police to hunt for him. The search was soon halted by the Second Front, the Allied landings on the Normandy beaches in June, 1944. It wasn't until August 24, when Paris was liberated, did the newspapers feel free to tell their readers about the mass murders carried out by Marcel Petiot.

For several days they splashed the story on their front pages, described the grisly finds in the private hospital, and ran interviews with his relatives and friends. Georgette stoutly affirmed that he was a patriot and those people he had been forced to liquidate had been traitors of France. She was a lone voice. Everybody else was certain that he had been an exterminator for the Germans and would be found hiding somewhere in Germany when the Allies arrived there.

There was one other voice clanging in Petiot's defence, one lone voice which attracted immediate attention and suspicion. The newspaper *Resistance* received a letter from somebody signing himself as "A still serving officer of the Resistance." "Petiot a

traitor?" he queried and hastened to add: "Not so. There is no
Frenchman more loyal than Marcel Petiot." The writer reminded
the editor of *Resistance* that Petiot had spent many months in a
Gestapo prison, and while he was there the Germans had used
his private hospital as a dumping ground for patriotic Frenchmen
whom they had shot. They had then sent the fire brigade and the
police to find the bodies before Petiot could clean up the place as
they wished Petiot to be blamed for their crimes. The motive,
the writer declared, was to have a big fuss made in the newspapers to detract attention from the defeats the Wehrmacht was
facing on the eastern front.

Petiot, declared the officer, was a great French patriot and
should be honoured. Soon everybody would see this clearly
when the war was over and the truth was revealed.

The editor, deciding it had been written by Petiot or another
lunatic just like him, hurried the letter to the police.

Freed from the heavy hampering arm of the German Army,
the Sûreté moved fast. The handwriting in the letter was checked
against that of officers who had enlisted in the newly-formed
French Army in Paris. The handwriting was found to resemble
that of a Captain Henri Valéry, who was serving with a battalion
at Reuilly. He had been in the army six weeks. They called at his
camp, a detention centre for prisoners, and found that he was
away. The captain specialised in the interrogation of both
German prisoners and other suspicious people, the police were
told, and so they spoke to his secretary. She was pretty Mlle
Cécile Dylma, aged twenty-five, who seemed to be a little on the
nervous side as if she had been badly frightened recently.
Hesitantly she admitted that the captain was very much a gentleman, but she quickly added, "He does have some peculiarly
sadistic habits." It appears that as if to prove he was very much
anti-German he would thump a broken-down enemy soldier
before the man could get the answer to his question out.

Petiot had changed his appearance. He now wore a luxuriant
beard, and the girl gave them an exact description of the captain,
as if she hoped he would be arrested very soon.

The police tracked him to the suburbs at Rue Faubourg St
Denis. They heard rumours of a heavily hirsute lunatic who was
in the habit of standing bare-chested at a window. There had
already been several complaints made to the local police. It was
while they were checking out the description of this Tarzan in
order to see if he was their man that the suspect was seen hurrying
out of the nearby Métro. He said when he was apprehended, "Do
hurry with your questions. There is a war on, you know. I'm
needed at the battlefield."

Asked about the remains in the cellar which totalled up to twenty-four bodies, Petiot corrected his questioners. He had kept a careful mental record, he said, and there was twenty-seven. He thought, all told, he had put down sixty-three people, and added, "They were all traitors to France, of course."

Who were Petiot's superiors? he was next asked. With the Germans gone, Petiot saw no reason why he shouldn't tell them, and he reamed off five names.

The five were all famous members of the Resistance. But, as Petiot well knew, they were dead. Another Gallic shrug. He reminded the detectives that he had been a prisoner of the Gestapo and that he had served in the Army in the first world war. He had re-enlisted in the Free French forces on September 27, a month after the Germans had been cleared from Paris.

What had happened to his police dossier at Villeneuve, which was missing? Again a Gallic shrug from Petiot. Why should he know since he had left the confounded place in 1930?

It was said that Petiot was never short of an answer and he loved an audience. When it was pointed out that some of the remains in the pit seemed to be of children, Petiot was baffled for perhaps a second, and then the answer: "I cannot remember any children collaborators but there were some men of very small stature – midgets."

It was eighteen months before Petiot stood trial. It lasted three weeks. Petiot sat to attention like a cocker-spaniel not wanting to miss a thing, as an army of relatives solemnly came to court and told how they had last seen a missing father, husband, brother or son when he had gone off to Monsieur Petiot's private hospital, to begin a journey out of France.

Again and again it was pointed out that if these men had got through as Petiot claimed they had, why hadn't their relatives in France heard from them. France had been freed. Paris had been liberated in August 1944 and this was now March 1946, so why had none of these people returned or even written to their loved ones?

A leader of the Resistance appeared and was questioned on Petiot's knowledge of Resistance matters. He showed that the only things Petiot knew about the Resistance was common gossip from the boulevards and what he had since read in the newspapers.

It was estimated that Petiot's profits from the murders ran into six figures, and his motive had been one of greed as well as sadistic gratification.

It took a jury of seven and three judges two and a half hours to find him guilty of twenty-four of the twenty-seven murders with which he was charged. The prosecution took no chances. They based their charge on how many bodies the remains totalled up to, not what Petiot's memory told him the number was.

There was a hubbub in court and the Judge had to repeat the findings. Petiot lost his temper on hearing that he had been found guilty and sentenced to death. He yelled obscenities at the judge, called him a traitor, maintained that the dead bodies had been the remains of German soldiers and that he, practically alone, had waged total war on the German Army of Occupation. Finding that the judge wasn't listening, Petiot swung on his guards, like a Tarzan, and began to throw punches at them. "I deserve a medal, not the guillotine," he called out over and over again.

It is probable that Petiot was neither pro-German nor anti-Semetic. His motives: profit and sexual perversion. These tendencies, but for the war, would probably have remained hidden. But in the chaotic conditions following the Occupation he saw vast opportunities. People could disappear without questions being asked. It would be assumed that wealthy refugees had escaped to England or America or been taken prisoner by the Gestapo. He decided to murder rich refugees whose relatives wouldn't raise an alarm because they thought Petiot, at some risk to himself, had helped smuggle them from the country. Petiot not only made a huge profit and got a sexual kick out of seeing them on their way, but became a hero in the eyes of the trusting relatives who remained behind.

He had some twenty banking accounts to "lose" his ill-gotten gains in, and if he thought that exposure might come one day he never gave it a thought. Perhaps he was much too busy to think. People who remember him recall that he put in a hard day's work at the Rue Caumartin surgery, and possibly, with the Germans in Paris and the great advances they were making in Russia, Petiot thought that he would never be discovered.

The Little Exterminator went to the guillotine on May 26 1946, confident, with a smirk which was almost a giggle on his wan cheeks. It was the same giggle that he would have employed at least sixty-seven times, while looking through the spyhole in the garage at Rue Lesueur, watching his victims scratch their lives away.

DR. HERMANN SANDER

Every book should have a hero, and if this work must have one, the OBVIOUS candidate is Dr. Hermann Sander, of New Hampshire, U.S.A., who stood trial for the alleged murder of a patient in 1950. The prosecution produced no motive at the trial, which saw Dr. Sander found not guilty. The newspapers described it as a mercy killing and it aroused world-wide interest and controversy at the time, and brought scores of reporters to Manchester, New Hampshire, to report every wrinkle of the affair.

Between the arrest of the doctor and the trial, all the arguments for and against euthanasia were aired, but what obviously gave the story its massive world audience appeal was the fact that it aptly showed the stress and distress doctors face in dealing with patients. Dr. Sander had nursed Mrs. Abbie Borroto, aged 59, for nearly a year and was a daily witness to the magnificient fight she was putting up for her life. But during that time, in which he had seen her weight reduced by half, he had been forced to live with the fact that there could be only one outcome. Mrs. Borroto's cancer would eventually kill her.

It was a long, painful and wasting illness. And anybody witnessing the patient's fight for life and the courage she showed, would have been inhuman if he did anything other but become involved. It was a case, therefore, and these must be common, where a witness suffered almost as much as the patient. When death for Mrs. Borroto seemed imminent, indeed might already medically have taken place, Dr. Sander injected air into her vein. He next, matter of factly, told a nurse that it was all over now for the patient. Then, with a characteristic honesty which people had come to expect from him, Dr. Sander recorded what he had done in his notes on the case, and left them with a nurse-secretary for typing. The girl saw the statement that air had been injected into the patient and reported the matter immediately to the hospital management.

Dr. Sander heard a rumour that the management was consulting with the police on the matter, but went about his duties as usual during that Christmas week in 1949. On December 29, two police detectives arrested him on first degree murder, which automatically carried the death sentence.

Dr. Sander, who was born just across the border in Canada, was 41. He was of small build, walked with a slight stoop and had a sallow complexion. He reminded some people of an absent-minded professor. Although he didn't look like the Hollywood conception of a hero, Dr. Sander was already one for many people in the community. He worked harder than most doctors, and he never thought of picking up his fee if the patient looked as if he couldn't afford it. He always put his work first and neglected worldly pleasures. Committed to his fellow man by an idealistic zeal, Sander was obviously the kind of doctor who had strong convictions. But with equally strong emotions, he was of the type who would let them at some stage rule his reason. It is these types of men who make saints and martyrs, but they also shake mountains and change the world. Why Dr. Sander did what he did, he couldn't explain, not even to himself. Mrs. Borroto was undoubtedly suffering and, if alive, hanging on to life by a thread. Emotionally wrought up by her appearance, Dr. Sander undoubtedly acted on impulse.

The case against euthanasia, even voluntarily when the sufferer makes the decision is, I believe, an unanswerable one. It is realistic and rational, of course, and not emotional. The paramount consideration for many people, especially the residents of New Hampshire, who were predominantly Catholic at the time, was religious. Murder or suicide, which euthanesia involves, is the dreadful sin. But there are other, more earthy, more practical grounds for rejecting euthanasia than the moral and religious ones. It could be argued that such a decision shouldn't be left to the sufferer who, while undergoing stress of body and mind, is in no condition to give a clear judgement. If, alternatively, the decision should be decided by a doctor, or a committee of doctors, why should they bear the responsibility for making such an irrevocable move? Moreover, by his oath, a doctor is instructed to preserve life, not take it, so why should he go in direct opposition to his Hippocratic oath? There are sound medical objections too. The cure which will save the sufferer might not be on hand at the moment, but new medical discoveries are being made, and the cure could be just around the corner. Another medical fact, disquieting but true, is that doctors don't always know when a patient has an incurable disease or when, and if, it will kill.

Time and time again in the cases mentioned in this book, doctors have displayed baffled ignorance in dealing with patients, and death certificates and in their testimony given in court.

With the better facilities and medical knowledge available today doctors are more likely to be right than wrong, but they still make mistakes – mistakes through lack of knowledge or human error.

The British Department of Health showed recently how common these errors were when they checked the reasons given for death on several hundred death certificates, against the findings of post mortems in each case. They discovered that only sixty per cent of the doctors had diagnosed the correct cause of death. Dr. Hubert Trowell, who carried out an investigation for the British Medical Association into euthanasia, has said, "I often found in post mortems that the cancer which everybody thought had killed the subject, wasn't there."

Dr. Trowell is against euthanasia – as are most doctors. If it was legal to kill, he declared, all sorts of pressures would be brought on doctors and patients. Aged patients would face a crippling sort of blackmail. They might feel, like the old usually do, that they don't wish to be a burden to anybody, relatives and hospitals alike. They might believe, because of their age, that they are in their last illness when in fact they have only a minor complaint which, once cured will leave them with another ten, twenty, or even thirty years of life.

The only person who should, if euthanasia was acceptable, be allowed to rescind his life is the patient, but if undergoing a painful illness, the patient's resolve could be at low ebb. Many diseases drive the sick into a low degree of melancholia in which they have the wish to die. This is the time when, if euthansia was legal, they might very well sign their life away.

Depressive psychosis is a common disease, and a feature of it is that the patient desires his own death. But this suicide urge goes immediately on recovery. In Britain, some 600 people suffer spinal cord injuries each year, and eight out of ten of these, in the first few black days, express the wish to commit suicide. After six months however, and having conditioned themselves to a new way of life, only one in ten wishes to end it all. Doctors agree that they shouldn't take life, nor be responsible for taking it. What they do agree to do, however, is not prolong life by drug or surgery if life is obviously moving to its end, or if life will cease to be meaningful for the patient. Their duty, therefore, becomes the simple one of ensuring that the patient doesn't suffer any more pain than can be helped in the final stages. Doctor's won't save a patient who is obviously going to be a helpless vegetable, but they will reduce pain by increasing the morphine injections and might, possibly, carry out an operation to neutralise the nervous system in order to keep a patient comfortable until the end. But an increase of morphine injections doesn't, as some people believe, gradually kill the patient. It might get the patient "hooked" on the drug, but it won't kill. An over-dose of morphine would be fourteen times the amount a terminal patient would receive.

These were the arguments for and against euthanasia which were heatedly debated in the United States when Dr. Sander was charged with the first degree murder of Mrs. Abbie Borroto. The facts given at the trial were these. Over the Christmas period, when people had been celebrating the holiday of brotherly love, Dr. Sander had bent over Mrs. Borroto's bed in a private room in Hillsborough County Hospital. It was almost impossible to detect life in the patient. If death had not already taken place, it could only be a matter of minutes or hours away. The nurse tried, unsuccessfully, to find a pulse beat. Then Dr. Sander turned to the patient again, this time with a syringe. He made an injection, and told the nurse that Mrs. Borroto, their patient for a year, had gone. After he had noted the fact that he had injected air into the patient he calmly passed the notes for typing to the secretary. What particularly concerned this woman was that an injection of air into a vein had, traditionally, been a method of murder in fictional detective stories.

Supposedly, the air reaches the heart in much the same way as a blood clot, causing a blockage and thus stoppage and heart failure. This theory, beloved of thriller writers, (and believed by this nurse), became a controversial issue at the trial. Again medical men made a spectacle of themselves in court, one group maintaining air does kill, another group that it couldn't possibly do so. But if the latter were right, what did Dr. Sander believe? And what was the point of the injection?

When he was arrested, the doctor was busy in his surgery. He was perky and confident and told his assistant not to cancel any of his appointments. He told the two detectives that he had been expecting them. He also said that he gave the injection as an act of charity and added, "The family asked me if I could do anything to end her suffering."

Although the charge was murder, and in the first degree, Dr. Sander's confidence had not been wrong. He was allowed out on bail, which hadn't been given in a first degree murder charge since the days of the Chicago gangsters. It was a stiff bail, $25,000, but Dr. Sander had many friends and the sum was forthcoming. Immediately, Dr. Sander won support from almost every walk of life. But legally, and there were no excuses permitted, Dr. Sander had murdered, claimed the state. The law made no allowances for mercy killing. As far as William Phinney, the state's attorney-general, was concerned, Dr. Sander had committed premeditated and wilful murder. Although they had been schoolchums and life-long friends, Mr. Phinney let it be known that he would prosecute the case with the full vigour of the law.

Mr. Phinney had local support, for although Dr. Sander was popular, two thirds of the population were Catholic. Some people thought that some of the doctor's remarks to the press, if he indeed made them, were arrogant, and in the circumstances, obnoxious. On the matter of the injections, he was alleged to have told reporters: "Doctors tell me this has happened many times but are never put in the record. My mistake, it is said, was that I put it in the record. They say I'm a couple of decades ahead of my time."

It seemed, to Catholics, that Dr. Sander was crowing over his courage and visualising a time, not too far ahead, when euthanasia would be legal. Members of the Borroto family also took different sides. The husband, Reginald Borroto, saddened by the charge, described Dr. Sander as "the biggest man I've ever met", and while one of Mrs. Borroto's brothers said he "bore the doctor no ill will," two others came out against him because, they said, the decision was God's, and they reminded the world that Mrs. Borroto, by her fight, had refused to give up the struggle.

A dramatic shock came at the preliminary hearing in the nearby city of Manchester, where the prosecution charged that the doctor had injected ten cubic centimetres of air four times into the patient.

Hitherto, people thought there had been just one injection given on the spur of the moment, but here was the prosecution saying the doctor had made four separate injections. For a time, the doctor's supporters were shaken, but they had rallied round by the time of trial proper. The doctor was released on the same bail as before and a post mortem on Mrs. Borroto was called for.

The biggest problem at the trial, which opened on February 20, was finding a jury which would suit both sides. It took two full court days, in which some two hundred candidates were questioned and rejected by both prosecution and defence, before the trial started. The attorney-general, Mr. Phinney, had watered down his case somewhat. Opening for the prosecution, he said that forty centimetres of air, injected into a woman in Mrs. Borroto's weak condition, would *probably* have caused her death. Mr. Phinney also stated now that the state wouldn't press for the death sentence. One phrase was missing on both sides – mercy killing. Mr. Phinney refused to put forward any motive why Dr. Sander should kill Mrs. Borroto. He merely stated that he had committed the crime. Mr. Phinney had no intention of allowing an emotive phrase like "mercy killing" into court and, seemingly, also the defence was against the phrase being used.

The court simply ignored this motive which all the world was discussing, and which had brought Dr. Sander 3,000 letters of sympathy. It also brought writers like John O'Hare and Fannie Hurst into court to write about the trial.

The defence immediately tried to establish that Mrs. Borroto was already dead when the defendant made the injections. It seems that another doctor, Dr. Albert Snay, had pronounced Mrs. Borroto dead before Dr. Sander had even arrived. The nurse who witnessed the injections, Miss Josephine Connor, told the court that Dr. Sander had described the patient as "practically moribund" on the day before the injections and that on the following day, Mrs. Borroto had died ten minutes after the injections.

She also gave her version of a talk which took place between Dr. Sander and Dr. Robert Biron, the county medical referee after the injections had been reported. She said Dr. Biron asked Dr. Sander if he knew he had broken the law and she quoted Dr. Sander as replying, "Yes, I have broken the law before, and I have been through stop signs." Dr. Biron retorted that this was more serious than traffic offences for this was murder, and to this, the nurse said, Dr. Sander had answered that he realised he had broken the law but that the law should be changed. Dr. Biron had responded by saying, "Why didn't you change it first before you did this?"

According to Nurse Connor, Dr. Biron also asked Dr. Sander if he realised the seriousness of the situation, and to this, she quoted him as replying, that he thought the Medical Association would probably reprimand him for it and tell him not to do it again. There might well have been a personality clash between Dr. Biron and Dr. Sander of some standing, but even so, if Nurse Connor's evidence was sound, Dr. Sander's levity didn't sit well with the public. It was thought to be both dogmatic and arrogant.

The attorney-general, Mr. Phinney, deftly established for the jury that Mrs. Borroto was alive at the time of the injections. This occured when he cross-examined another nurse, Miss Elizabeth Rose, who had also attended the patient. Miss Rose said three people had been unable to detect a pulse beat before Dr. Sander arrived and gave the injections. Another nurse, besides herself, couldn't find a pulse beat, and she had called in Dr. Albert Snay, who happened to be passing the room, and asked for his opinion. He had tried for a pulse, also failed, and then tried for a heart beat with his stethoscope. But, Miss Rose admitted, Dr. Snay hadn't pronounced the patient dead. Then Dr. Sander had arrived. The two doctors had conferred but Nurse Rose said she hadn't heard what they were saying.

After Dr. Snay then left, testified the nurse, Dr. Sander now tried to find a pulse. He didn't tell her whether he found it or not but asked her for a syringe. She had handed him an empty one, which he had applied to the patient. Then, under Mr. Phinney's questions Nurse Rose said, "I heard a gasp from Mrs. Borroto, and then Dr. Sander turned to me and said 'Air in the veins will act like an embolus.'" She described the doctor's actions, the plunger going down on the empty syringe connected to the patient's arm and which remained down for two or three minutes. Afterwards, Dr. Sander handed her the syringe and needle and told her he would notify the family and call the undertaker.

Mr. Phinney, by elucidating that the patient had gasped, thereby established the fact that she had been alive. Mention of the "embolus", a bubble of air racing to the heart, showed, if Nurse Rose's evidence was correct, what the doctor had in mind by making the injections.

Dr. Sander's followers rebounded from this setback, however, when Mr. Borroto testified. Initially he had favoured the prosecution, for he denied telling Dr. Sander at any time that he would like his wife's life terminated so as to end her fruitless suffering. But then, in reference to Dr. Sander, he said, "I couldn't feel any more affection or kindness towards him even if he was my own brother. If my wife had been the doctor's mother or sister he couldn't have done more to minister to her than he did." He added that during her stay at the hospital, Dr. Sander had done her many kindnesses. He had brought her several gifts, including a canary, which had given her many hours of pleasure.

Dr. Albert Snay testified that he had examined Mrs. Borroto before Dr. Sander arrived and added, "I concluded she was dead and I remarked to Miss Rose that the patient seemed to be gone. Dr. Sander arrived and I said something to the effect that there was nothing to be done." Dr. Snay hadn't reported the matter elsewhere because she was Dr. Sander's patient. He added: "From her appearance, it was amazing to me she had lived as long as she did. Nothing Dr. Sander or anyone else could have done would have affected her condition."

Dr. Robert Biron's evidence, as medical referee, was most damaging. He began by quoting the record Dr. Sander had made – "patient given ten c.c. of air, repeated four times, and expired ten minutes after this was started." His evidence remained unchanged as that given by the nurse who had witnessed the conversation. Dr. Sander had told him that he had permission from the Borroto family and that if he had broken the law, the law should be changed.

Two doctors who had carried out the post mortem gave details. A Dr. Miller said he found death had been caused by pulmonary embolism – a blood clot in the lungs; the second, Dr. Milton Helpern, deputy medical examiner for New York City, confirmed this but gave more details. "A big bubble of air," he said, would as effectively block circulation as "a big clot of blood." While the autopsy couldn't, of course, determine the presence of air, Dr. Helpern though it was "significant that the autopsy didn't reveal any other cause of death which would have caused as rapid a death."

There it was then, the implication that but for the injection, Mrs. Borroto might have lived for some considerable time yet. Before introducing their own witnesses, and ignoring all that had gone before, the defence cheekily asked that the case be dismissed on the grounds that the prosecution had failed to show that the death had been caused by a felony. Having failed to get this, the defence went all out to gain as much sympathy for Dr. Sander as they could. Emotion is permitted to be more a weapon in American courts than in English ones, the latter being more concerned with facts than why's and wherefores. These can always be considered later when the degree of punishment is made to fit the crime.

The defence now attempted to show why Dr. Sander had made the injections. It was because of the stresses and strains of modern life, they said. But like the prosecution before them, they pulled up short before introducing that emotive phrase – "mercy killing."

The jury, of course, would know the phrase – for nothing else had been more debated for the last couple of months in the state than the alleged mercy killing of Mrs. Borroto by Dr. Sander. The prosecution, however, didn't want to see the phrase introduced into court in case it created too much sympathy for the doctor, and thus an acquittal, while the jury blithely ignored the facts. The defence didn't want it introduced because it gave the jury a motive as to why the doctor might kill his patient, and, although they might be deeply sympathetic, they would be forced to do their duty by the law as it existed and find him guilty.

Defence witnesses included Mrs. Borroto's daughter who vouchsafed that the doctor had felt as badly as she had about her mother's death. After the death, Dr. Sander had invited her and her father to come and stay at his house "not overnight or for a day, but for a week or as long as we wanted to."

The doctor's secretary, Helen Maciolek, testified that Dr

Sander was no ordinary doctor. "He was a saint," she said. "He was a twenty-four hour doctor who never took a proper day off. He was always available when other doctors were not."

Whether Dr. Sander was a saint or a devil wasn't the point under debate. It was whether he had murdered Mrs. Borroto or not, and if so, was it by accident or by design.

So a long succession of witnesses came forward to testify on the doctor's saintly qualities. The court was told of the clinic he had founded for under-privileged children, of the $6,000 he had collected for a new hospital wing and of how he allowed poor patients to convalesce at his home. In fact so popular was he that $11,000 had been raised locally for help in his defence.

Having established this, the defence got back to the case. It was as if they were suddenly aware of the fact that while their client might be God-like in his selflessness, it didn't give him a legal right to play God. They introduced several witnesses, all nurses, who testified that in their opinion Mrs. Borroto was indeed dead before Dr. Sander gave the injections. And then they called on Dr. Sander to take the stand.

If some of the man's reported statements in the press had seemed arrogant, he certainly didn't look arrogant or cocksure in court. Throughout the long hearing he presented a picture of a man who had suffered much and was still suffering. Dark rings around his eyes bespoke sleepless nights. It was noticed too that he avoided any face to face confrontation with his old friend, Mr. Phinney, the attorney-general.

However, he was calm and relaxed as he testified. He had decided to become a doctor, he said, after reading a novel called *The Magnificent Obsession*. His wife complained that he overworked, but he lived for his practice. He became choked with emotion as he described Mrs. Borroto's final days. For the last two weeks of her life, he testified, she had been unable to move, and the amount of food she had eaten during the last month was hardly adequate enough to make up a normal-sized meal. "In her last week," he said, "she looked like a dead person."

He described the moment of the injections in a distraught and baffled manner. "It was my opinion then that she was dead. I can't explain exactly what action I took then. Something snapped. Why I did it, I can't tell. It doesn't make sense." He denied agreeing to kill Mrs. Borroto or having any intention to carry out such an action. He added, "I don't know what I intended to do with the syringe. I remember trying to get it into her vein, and I didn't use a tournique to bring up the vein. Her veins were collapsed."

Saying that there was no blood on Mrs. Borroto's arm and that he had used a ten centimetre syringe, Dr. Sander added, "I withdrew the plunger to make suction, but nothing came out. There was no blood. I injected a couple of cubic centimetres, and I then injected a couple more. Nothing happened. There was a slight swelling around the needle. I continued to inject small amounts of air until the entire ten cubic c.c. was gone. During the procedure there was no indication of life, no reaction," he added.

Dr. Sander admitted making further injections. "I detached the syringe by holding the needle with my left hand and unscrewing the syringe. I repeated the process with five or six cubic centimetres, at two centimetres at a time, until the syringe was empty." He said that this brought no change in her appearance nor did she give any reaction at all, and he then repeated the injection a third time. Altogether he thought that he had injected between twenty-five and twenty-eight centimetres of air, not the forty the prosecution claimed. Asked why he had made a confession in the records, which had led to his arrest, Dr. Sander said calmly, "I think it is the duty of every doctor to put down on the charts what he has done for every patient, whether it has any effect or not."

Dr. Sander also said he was probably not being fair to himself when he stipulated in the records that death had come within ten minutes. "It was casual dictation," he said. "The fact that I say she expired at that time doesn't mean she died at that time. It's merely a means of closing out the case on the chart."

The prosecution now hammered Dr. Sander, but the only admission he would make during his four hour ordeal was that his action with the syringe had been "irrational behaviour."

The doctor admitted, under this weight of questioning, that he had been influenced in his action by Mrs. Borroto's appearances. He said, "It was the expression on her face, the long suffering, and also the suffering of her husband. Her expression touched me off. What I did, doesn't make sense. I don't know why I put the needle into her vein."

He re-affirmed his conviction, however, that he hadn't taken Mrs. Borroto's life. He stressed, "I told the authorities I hadn't taken a life, nor committed a crime, and I meant by that that I hadn't taken a life. The whole action was irrational behaviour." Pursued relentlessly by Mr. Phinney, Dr. Sander claimed; "I knew I hadn't committed a sin. My conscience had been clear throughout the whole affair. I don't know why I did all these things. I was upset to do this, and I don't know why I kept on, nor why I stopped."

"Was Mrs. Borroto unconscious at the time of the injection?"
Mr. Phinney asked.

Dr. Sander promptly answered: "I knew she was dead."

"Yet you had this obsession to pump air into this poor dead soul?"

"That's right," Dr. Sander answered.

"Have you ever been of the opinion that a patient might be better served by being dead?"

"I have never thought that," said Dr. Sander, who also said he couldn't remember saying that he might have broken the law when first asked about the injections.

And now, as if the trial was a giant club sandwich, the defence introduced another dollop of character witnesses. Mrs. Sander confessed in the witness box that she had never wished to marry a doctor because they placed work before their families. She, however, had come to admire Dr. Sander. This had happened while they both worked in a New Jersey hospital. She had liked the respect that he had had for the poorer patients who came to the hospital. After they were married, she testified, she was never permitted to tell patients the doctor wasn't at home, whatever the time and no matter how tired he might be.

There were shades of Sir Philip Sydney when Nurse Gertrude Morency told the court that the doctor had given his own blood to a patient because, she said, "He said they need it more than I do."

Having again established their client sympathetically before the jury, the defence now launched the secret weapon they had nursed throughout the prolonged trial – the powerful mustard for the sandwich. It could have come straight out of Perry Mason. And it was going to take the shape once more of that old tug-of-war between medical men.

Earlier, two prosecution witnesses, both eminent doctors, had testified that their autopsy findings had shown them, most emphatically, that an injection of air had killed Mrs. Borroto. Now the defence produced Dr. Richard Ford, head of legal medicine at Harvard University. Dr. Ford, who is one of America's most celebrated pathologists, refuted the idea that the injections killed Mrs. Borroto. He had studied air embolism for nearly a year he said, and he found the argument between the prosecution and the defence pointless. Twenty-eight c.c.'s or forty c.c.'s of injected air made absolutely no difference to the patient, he maintained. In his considered opinion, the injection of forty c.c.'s of air would have the effect of only a small whisky.

Dr. Ford thought it would take between 200 and 300 c.c.'s of injected air to kill, and even then it would only be effective if introduced in the space of twenty-five seconds. He added that forty c.c.'s wasn't sufficient to block, appreciably, any part of the arterial system leading to the lung. The fact that a person's heart might be weak at the time of such an injection, he added, wouldn't make any difference.

In the United States, the law of *sub judice* doesn't apply and newspapers and commentators can remark on a trial while it is in progress. Earlier, newspapers had carried a front-page story in which Dr. Harry Robinson, of the University of Maryland Medical School, had announced his willingness to receive an injection of forty c.c.'s of air – now or at any time. He maintained vigorously, "Injections of air into the veins can't cause death."

The newspapers also quoted Dr. Robinson as saying that he himself had given air injections to his patients without results either "good or bad".

If the American jury didn't see Dr. Robinson's pronouncements – (because newspapers are clipped of any comment on the trial before being delivered to a jury in their hotel rooms) – they heard Dr. Ford's evidence a day or so later, and this was startling. Two eminent doctors had found embolism as the cause of death when they had attended Mrs. Borroto's post mortem. But Dr. Ford, for the defence, had also attended the autopsy, and he didn't think that air embolism had killed the patient or in fact that air injections, unless in the great amounts stated earlier, could cause death at all.

Once again, as in so many trials, the jury – and the judge – were being asked, without medical knowledge, to evaluate and decide which contradictory medical evidence was the truth. From the human aspect, the jury must already have been uneasy. The prosecution, of course, had by no means made out an airtight case against Dr. Sander, although his actions with the syringe had been strange. To a man, the jury were almost certainly against conviction. They knew there had been no malice in the doctor's motives, but on the contrary, they had been dictated by deep compassion.

It wasn't so much that the doctor had played a God, as his detractors claimed, but that he had not been God-like in his strength to be above, and detatched, from the sufferings of his patient.

The defence, undoubtedly, had scored brilliantly by keeping Dr. Ford's testimony to the end. The prosecution must have realised what was coming but could do nothing about it. Dr. Ford was one of the leading pathologist's in the United States, and his evidence obviously imfluenced the jury.

On the seventeenth day of the trial, the jury left the court to deliberate. It took them sixty-nine minutes to find Dr. Sander not guilty of both first and second degree murder.

But in the joy which followed, Dr. Sander's days in the wilderness were not yet over. He was barred from entering a Roman Catholic hospital and then the state revoked his licence to practice, because, they said, even if the injections were made after Mrs. Borroto's death, they were still reprehensible morally. Dr. Sander, however, was told he could apply for reinstatement in the summer. He did so and was allowed to continue his practice. The trial remains as an illuminating example of the anomalous situation caused when public sentiment and the law, in the name of the ultimate public good, go separate and contradictory ways.